The Language of Mental Health

Series Editors
Michelle O'Reilly
The Greenwood Institute
University of Leicester
Leicester, UK

Jessica Nina Lester
School of Education
Indiana University
Bloomington, IN, USA

This series brings together rich theoretical and empirical discussion at the intersection of mental health and discourse/conversation analysis. Situated broadly within a social constructionist perspective, the books included within this series will offer theoretical and empirical examples highlighting the discursive practices that surround mental health and make 'real' mental health constructs. Drawing upon a variety of discourse and conversation analysis perspectives, as well as data sources, the books will allow scholars and practitioners alike to better understand the role of language in the making of mental health.

We are very grateful to our expert editorial board who continue to provide support for the book series. We are especially appreciative of the feedback that they have provided on earlier drafts of this book. Their supportive comments and ideas to improve the book have been very helpful in our development of the text. They continue to provide support as we continue to edit the book series 'the language of mental health'. We acknowledge them here in alphabetical order by surname.

More information about this series at
http://www.palgrave.com/gp/series/15193

Camilla Lindholm · Melisa Stevanovic ·
Elina Weiste
Editors

Joint Decision Making in Mental Health

An Interactional Approach

palgrave
macmillan

Editors
Camilla Lindholm
Faculty of Information Technology
and Communication Sciences
Tampere University
Tampere, Finland

Melisa Stevanovic
Faculty of Social Sciences
University of Helsinki
Helsinki, Finland

Elina Weiste
The Finnish Institute
of Occupational Health
Helsinki, Finland

University of Helsinki
Helsinki, Finland

The Language of Mental Health
ISBN 978-3-030-43530-1 ISBN 978-3-030-43531-8 (eBook)
https://doi.org/10.1007/978-3-030-43531-8

Cover credit: oxygen/gettyimages

This Palgrave Macmillan imprint is published by the registered company Springer Nature Switzerland AG
The registered company address is: Gewerbestrasse 11, 6330 Cham, Switzerland

Contents

Notes on Contributors

Beth Angell is a dean and professor at the School of Social Work, Virginia Commonwealth University, USA. Her research focuses on behavioral health, particularly on serious mental illness and its intersection with substance abuse and criminal justice involvement.

Evrinomy Avdi is an associate professor in clinical psychology at the School of Psychology of the Aristotle University of Thessaloniki, Greece. Her research interests lie in applying discursive and narrative research to the study of the process of psychotherapy, as well as the experience of serious illness.

Galina B. Bolden is an associate professor in the Department of Communication at Rutgers University, USA. In her research, she uses conversation analysis to examine a variety of settings: ordinary conversations between family and friends, doctor–patient interactions conducted with the help of language interpreters, and interactions in mental health settings.

Katie Ekberg is a research fellow at the University of Queensland, Australia. Her research involves using conversation analysis to examine communication in health care interactions. Her previous research has involved examining client–practitioner communication in cognitive behavioral therapy sessions, calls on a cancer helpline, and audiology appointments with adults and children with hearing-impairment.

Jennifer R. Guzmán is an assistant professor in the Department of Anthropology at the State University of New York at Geneseo, NY, USA. She conducts research at the intersection of linguistic and medical anthropology. Her research in Chile and the United States examines provider-patient communication across a range of conventional, CAM/IM, and indigenous medical paradigms.

Alexa Hepburn is a research professor in the Department of Communication at Rutgers University, USA. Her research focuses on developing innovations in the use and development of conversation analytic methods. A major focus is to highlight limitations in more traditional social science perspectives on emotion and influence and support applied work in professional client encounters.

Shuya Kushida received his Ph.D. in human and environmental studies from Kyoto University and is currently a professor at Osaka Kyoiku University, Japan. His research interests include doctor–patient interaction, conversation analysis, and sociology.

Amanda LeCouteur is an associate professor in psychology at the University of Adelaide, Australia, where she teaches in the fields of gender, social interaction, and philosophy of science. She has published in the areas of racism, education, gender, and health, and her current research involves analysis of interaction in helpline, medical, and counseling settings.

Vasileia Lerou is a Ph.D. candidate in the Psychology Department of Aristotle University of Thessaloniki, and a clinical psychologist. Her research interests are focused on dialogical perspectives in psychotherapy, nonverbal expression in clinical practice, and qualitative research. She practices psychology working with vulnerable social groups in humanitarian organizations.

Camilla Lindholm is a professor in Nordic languages at Tampere University, Finland. Her main research areas are interaction in institutional settings, and asymmetric interaction involving participants with communication impairments. She takes a special interest in applying her research findings in a dialogue with society.

F. Alethea Marti is a postdoctoral researcher at UCLA's Center for Health Services and Society (USA). Her research interests include discourse and narrative analysis, families' development of understandings about mental health care, and cultural and linguistic communication issues for Limited English Proficiency immigrant parents.

Michael McCreary has been involved in the development, implementation and evaluation of mental health interventions at UCLA's Center for Health Services and Society (USA) since 2011. He obtained his B.A. in history from UCLA and a master's degree in public policy from USC in 2011.

Lisa Mikesell is associate professor in the Department of Communication and associate faculty at the Institute for Health, Health Care Policy and Aging Research at Rutgers University, USA. With a focus on neurological and psychiatric disorders, she studies practices of patient engagement in community and clinic contexts to provide an ecological lens on everyday functioning and person-centered communication.

Jenny Paananen is a postdoctoral researcher at the University of Helsinki, Finland. In her research, she combines multimodal conversation analysis with interactional linguistics to explore co-operational resources and social involvement in institutional interaction.

Melisa Stevanovic is a senior university lecturer in sociology at the University of Helsinki, Finland. She has conducted a long series of studies on collaborative decision-making in both naturally occurring interaction at the workplace and in experimental settings. She has also published on the topic of interactional deficits and experiences of interaction.

Taina Valkeapää has master's degree in sociology and works as a research coordinator at the University of Helsinki, Finland. She has a background in social counseling, and as a trained sociologist she uses conversation analysis to study interactions involving individuals with intellectual disabilities and mental health problems.

Kaisa Valkia has a master's degree in social psychology and has conducted research on mental health rehabilitation and positioning at the University of Helsinki, Finland.

Elina Weiste is sociologist and a specialist researcher at the Finnish Institute of Occupational Health. She has a background as an occupational therapist in psychiatric rehabilitation and has extensive knowledge of individuals with mental illness and their training in social skills. Her recent projects include "Social and health care professionals as experts on client involvement" (European Social Fund 2019–2021).

Yuriko Yamakawa got her M.D. and Ph.D. from the University of Tsukuba, Japan and is currently a professor at Ibaraki Prefectural University of Health Sciences. Her research interests include psychiatry, mental health, and rehabilitation psychology.

Bonnie T. Zima is a child psychiatrist and health services researcher. Her research focuses on the unmet need for mental health services among high-risk child populations and the quality of mental health care for children enrolled in Medicaid-funded outpatient programs.

Transcription Symbols

[ ]	Overlapping talk
=	Latching
(.)	Micro pause
(0.1)	Timed pause
-	Cut-off of preceding sound
:	Extension of a sound
°word°	Quieter voice
WORD	Louder voice
>word<	Faster talk
<word>	Slower talk
£word£	Smiley voice
#word#	Creaky voice
.hh	Aspiration
hh	Out breath
word	Emphasis
w(h)ord(h)	Laugh particles
↑↓	Rise or fall in pitch
?	Rising intonation
!	Animated tone
,	Continuing intonation

¿	Pitch rise stronger than comma but weaker than question mark
.	Falling intonation
(---)	Transcriber could not hear what was said
((sitting))	Transcriber's descriptions of phenomena
↑___↑	Beginning, end and duration of multimodal actions
doc |	Identified participant's multimodal actions

Abbreviations

1, 2	Person
ABL	Ablative
ADE	Adessive
ADV	Adverb
AUX	Auxiliary verb
C	Copula verb "be"
CLI	Clitic
COMP	Comparative
COND	Conditional
CP	Conjunctional particle
ELA	Elative
ESS	Essive
FP	Final particle
GEN	Genitive
ILL	Illative
IMP	Imperative
INE	Inessive
INF	Infinitive
ITJ	Interjection
LK	Nominal linking particle

N	Nominalizer
NEG	Negation
OP	Object particle
P	Particle
PAR	Partitive
PASS	Passive
PL	Plural
POSS	Possessive suffix
PPC	Past participle
PPPC	Passive past participle
PST	Past tense
Q	Question (clitic) particle
QP	Quotative particle
SP	Subject particle
TP	Topic particle
TRA	Translative

Singular, third person, nominative, active and *present tense* are forms that have been considered unmarked. These have not been glossed.

List of Figures

1

Introduction: Social Inclusion as an Interactional Phenomenon

Elina Weiste, Melisa Stevanovic, and Camilla Lindholm

Social inclusion and exclusion are successful buzzwords in today's political discourse. At their core, these concepts were created to explain and help to transform the complex reality of our times. Famously, according to the citizenship theory by Marshall (1964), one of the more significant master trends in modern social change is movement toward increasing social inclusion (Colomy & Brown, 1996). The notion of social inclusion has been associated with various dimensions related to the basic needs of humans: occupation, protection, recognition, education, bonds, and participation (Canal, 2010, p. 15). Social exclusion, in contrast, has been

E. Weiste (✉) · M. Stevanovic
University of Helsinki, Helsinki, Finland
e-mail: elina.weiste@ttl.fi

M. Stevanovic
e-mail: melisa.stevanovic@helsinki.fi

C. Lindholm
Tampere University, Tampere, Finland
e-mail: camilla.lindholm@tuni.fi

C. Lindholm et al. (eds.), *Joint Decision Making in Mental Health*,
The Language of Mental Health, https://doi.org/10.1007/978-3-030-43531-8_1

defined as "refusing people and/or social groups' access to the resources which, in a specific place and at a specific historical time, are considered socially valuable and necessary for a dignified and autonomous life" (Canal, 2010, p. 10). While there are many causes of social exclusion, one of the factors repeatedly shown to lead to social exclusion is mental illness, which may hinder people in developing themselves in accordance with their wishes and abilities (e.g., Knapp, 2003; Morgan, Burns, Fitzpatrick, Pinfold, & Priebe, 2007; Payne, 2006). Even today, people with mental illnesses are in one of the most marginalized positions in society (WHO, 2013).

Participation is a key dimension of social inclusion—and one that we particularly seek to increase understanding of in this volume. Participation is an element of democratic citizenship that enables citizens to actively shape their social and economic circumstances (Pateman, 1970). In this volume, however, we focus on participation taking place in face-to-face social encounters, with reference to what Erving Goffman (1983) called the "interaction order." In other words, we seek to get to the root of the preconditions and consequences of participation by unraveling the interactional processes that underlie what makes it possible. We presuppose that participation in any social or societal sphere presupposes social interaction, which in turn requires the capacity to coordinate with and make sense of others' actions. Thus, drawing on joint decision-making as a specific arena of social interaction, where the participants' collaborative management of the turn-by-turn sequential unfolding of interaction can have tangible consequences for the participants' social and economic circumstances, we seek to increase understanding of the specific vulnerabilities that individuals with mental illness have in this context.

Social Inclusion and Participation in Mental Health Care

Both social inclusion and participation are central notions in the contemporary discussion on social and health care services. Current international mental health policy recommendations emphasize the importance of client involvement, which means actions that support clients' willingness and ability to make independent decisions about their own lives and to take action to enhance their own well-being (Royal College of Psychiatrists Social Inclusion Scoping Group, 2009; WHO, 2013). In social and health care, social inclusion refers to the individual's sense of belonging within the community, and that he or she can influence issues affecting himself or herself and the surrounding environment (Sihvo et al., 2018). Social inclusion includes the right to be informed about issues relating to oneself, the opportunity to express one's opinion and contribute to the decisions concerning one's health and well-being (Sihvo et al., 2018). Social inclusion requires a feeling of meaningfulness, belonging to a whole, and the ability to form meaningful social relationships. The elements of social inclusion include both the right to participate in one's own care and opportunities to influence the planning and development of services (Sihvo et al., 2018).

From Professional Authority to Client Involvement

Even though mental health clients' opportunities for social inclusion remain weak in many respects (e.g., WHO, 2013), over the past few decades there have been significant changes in this regard. At the beginning of the 1900s, mental hospitals were the mainstream structures for the treatment of people with mental illnesses (Grob, 2014). Treatment decisions about hospital admission and discharge were made by professionals, often against the patient's own will. Since the 1940s the human rights movement gained more international influence, focusing attention on violations of basic human rights of patients in mental hospitals (Hänninen, 2012). The process of de-hospitalization that began in the 1950s led to the downsizing and closure of hospitals, reducing the number of hospital patients and leading to the development of different types of inpatient facilities (Grob, 2014). This trend was strongly influenced by the social psychiatry movement, which demanded respect for the agency of those suffering from mental illnesses and thereby shifted the focus from the ill individuals to the societal structures (Alanko & Hellman, 2017). At the same time, movements such as the antipsychiatry movement and the survivor and service user movements campaigned strongly for the patients' rights to self-determination (Alanko & Hellman, 2017). However, decision-making within mainstream psychiatry remained focused on the professionals' authority. Psychiatric professionals made decisions on the basis of medical knowledge, relying on what was deemed best for the patient without much of their involvement in the decision-making process (Charles, Gafni, & Whelan, 1997). The role of the patient was mainly restricted to expressing his or her consent to the professional's decision—consent that most often was not needed to implement the treatment decisions in practice. On the other hand, the expansion of psychiatric care to include, not only those seriously ill but also anyone suffering from mental health problems had resulted in a new group of individuals voluntary seeking access to treatment (Alanko & Hellman, 2017). Thus, mental health professionals had increasingly to respond to individuals' own perceptions of having a mental health problem, which necessitated treatment. This resulted in the service users starting to be seen as active agents, autonomously seeking help, rather than as passive, stigmatized patients, subjected to professionals' authoritative power (Alanko & Hellman, 2017).

In the 1980s, psychiatry was strongly influenced by the so-called "consumerist" movement with its members enforcing their role as consumers of mental health services (Rissmiller & Rissmiller, 2006). This movement did not seek to abolish the traditional mental health system, as was the aim in the antipsychiatry movements, but it did seek to increase the opportunities for patients to decide what services and treatments were most suitable for themselves (Rissmiller & Rissmiller, 2006). From a decision-making perspective, it became vital for professionals to provide patients with all the information needed for them to be able to decide on the most effective solution (Charles et al., 1997). The role of a professional became limited to providing the kind of medical information that a patient would not have access to without the professional's specialized expertise. At its most extreme, a professional should not give any recommendations for specific treatments, as they might reveal the professional's own views, which, in turn, could constrain the patient's ability to make his or her own decision (Rissmiller & Rissmiller, 2006). At the same time, mental health services were increasingly transferred to primary health care settings, and client-centeredness became a key guiding paradigm (Alanko & Hellman, 2017). Even today, client-centeredness is posited as the primary method of mental health service delivery (O'Donovan, 2007). The core idea of this model is to elicit and understand clients' experiential perspectives, feelings, concerns, expectations, needs, and functioning, in order to reach a shared understanding of the problem and its treatment (Epstein et al., 2005, p. 1517). The client-centered care philosophy emphasizes values of choice, self-determination, and empowerment, encouraging the client to form a collaborative partnership with the service provider (Epstein et al., 2005). These ideas represent a marked shift from the traditional asymmetric doctor–patient relationship, involving a passive patient and a dominant clinician (Roter, 2000).

Along with client-centeredness, there has been an increasing appreciation of expertise originating from first-hand experience of mental health problems (Alanko & Hellman, 2017). This "user expert" perspective originated from the user involvement movement, which was especially active in the UK in the late 1970s. User involvement generally means that they engage in the planning, development, and evaluation of social and health care services (Crawford et al., 2002). In addition to contributing to changes in the provision of services, user involvement can also be seen as valuable in itself (Osborne & Strokosch, 2013). Especially in mental health care, the clients' right to have a say in their own care has been considered as a central aspect of user involvement. In the current mental health policy statements, clients have the right to be heard and to consent to services in agreement with a professional (Royal College of Psychiatrists Social Inclusion Scoping Group, 2009). The mental health client also has the right to influence the design and implementation of the services provided for himself or herself, such as the development of a treatment plan. Contributing to plans about one's own treatment is not only considered as a right but also a prerequisite for successful service delivery (Tambuyzer, Pieters, & Van Audenhove, 2014). The starting assumption is that when participating, the client will take more responsibility for his or her situation, and will cope better on his or her own in the future (Tambuyzer et al., 2014).

Making Health Care Decisions Together

Clients' involvement in their own care is deeply anchored with the service users *participating in decision-making processes* (Thompson, 2007). By shifting the distribution of power from professionals to service users, the latter are seen to be empowered with greater influence over those decisions that affect them (see Alanko & Hellman, 2017). An especially important policy for the realization of the new distribution of power in this type of decision-making is the co-implication of the client in treatment decisions—a paradigm that is currently known as the "shared decision-making" model (SDM).

SDM is a collaborative process wherein both clinician and client are engaged to share information about preferences and values to reach consensus about treatment which they mutually agree to implement (Charles, Gafni, & Whelan, 1997). SDM was borne out of general medicine but the trend has been paralleled in mental health care in which it is considered as integral to a client-centered paradigm (Epstein et al., 2005). The SDM model recognizes that clients have important experiential knowledge of their illness and expertise over their personal values and preferences. They are also best equipped to know their treatment needs (Department of Health [DOH], 2001). Thus, clients are intended to focus on value-based aspects of treatment decision, whereas clinicians are assigned technical aspects of the decisions (Treichler & Spaulding, 2017).

Typical elements of decision-making in SDM involve describing a need for decision, describing options, exploring the client's values, negotiating a course of action, and making plans for follow-up (e.g., Volk et al., 2014). There are plenty of both generic and diagnosis-specific decision-support tools to aid the implementation of the SDM elements to clinical practice (see e.g., Option Grid: https://health.ebsco.com/products/option-grid). These tools may target behavior change in either clinicians or clients (Slade, 2017). For instance, in the case of depression, the use of these tools, in combination with clients obtaining information about client involvement, has led to an increased level of client participation and treatment satisfaction without lengthening the consultation time (Loh et al., 2007).

The SDM model has been argued to work well when the client's problem is relatively narrow, when no further client participation beyond actual treatment decision is needed, and when the client can choose from among several options that the clinicians have listed (Treichler & Spaulding, 2017). However, the model has been criticized for being inconsistent with the values of the so-called "recovery approach," which can be viewed as an overarching philosophy that encompasses the notions of self-determination, self-management, personal growth, empowerment, and choice (e.g., Anthony, 2007; Goossensen, Zijlstra, & Koopmanschap, 2007). From the perspective of the recovery approach, the SDM model involves a connotation that clinicians may choose *not* to share aspects of decision-making with the client, based on their clinical judgment of the client's ability to make the decision. The client is seen as too symptomatic to make the right choice (Treichler & Spaulding, 2017).

Use of the so-called "collaborative decision-making" (CDM) model has been proposed to avoid the limitations of the SDM model. CDM is a broader model of decision-making in mental health care, which is not restricted only to clinical treatment decisions. CDM is based on the idea of clients' and professionals' equal responsibility and power in decision-making processes (Treichler & Spaulding, 2017). In contrast to traditional decision-making models, which have little room for clients having varying needs and preferences, the CDM model highlights the personalized treatment processes. In the decision-making process, the clients and clinicians first share all relevant information on the client's needs and treatment options. Second, the client weighs the pros and cons of each option within the context of his or her individual needs. The clinician offers opinions without influencing the client's preferences, and above all, helps the client to reflect on what makes the best choice for him or her. Third, the client and the professional make a joint agreement based upon each person's understanding of what makes the most sense within the client's unique situation. Moreover, it is seen as crucial that decisions are open for continued reconsideration after the joint decision has been made. (Treichler & Spaulding, 2017). Similar to the SDM model, the CDM model has also led to an increasing number of aids, which aim to improve collaborative decision-making skills of clinicians and clients (e.g., Andrews, Drake, Haslett, & Munusamy, 2010).

One challenge in implementing decision-making models in the context of mental health care, especially in the case of severe mental illnesses, is the possibility that the capacities of a client's decision-making have been impaired due to deficits in cognitive processes, such as attention and executive functioning, or formation of preference (Ernst & Paulus, 2005). For instance, individuals with schizophrenia may have difficulties assigning affective value to the consequences of their decision (Larquet, Coricelli, Opolczynski, & Thibaut, 2010), which hampers the smoothness of decision-making processes. In addition, their deficits in integrating cognitive and emotional components of decision-making contribute to their inability to generate adaptive behaviors in social situations (Larquet et al., 2010)—a locus of complex interactional phenomena that this volume also seeks to illustrate.

While there is much knowledge about the deficits in the individual decision-making capacities in individuals with mental illnesses, this volume broadens the view about this phenomenon by investigating real-life interactional encounters in which people with mental health problems need to manage their participation in joint decision-making and when the social consequences of their conduct become apparent in the subsequent unfolding of interactions.

Joint Decision-Making as an Interactional Process

We will now proceed to describing joint decision-making as an interactional process. First, we will summarize the basic principles and assumptions of conversation analysis with a special regard to asymmetric interaction. Next, we will discuss conversation-analytic studies of joint decision-making in organizations, multiprofessional teams, and everyday encounters. Finally, we will consider joint decision-making in clinical encounters.

Conversation Analysis and the Study of Asymmetric Interaction

CA is a method to study naturally occurring interaction and its structures (Heritage, 1984). Rather than concentrating on the linguistic form or propositional content of talk, conversation analysis sets out to study what people do with talk, how talk is used to perform everyday actions (e.g., asking, requesting, telling, and complaining), and what the consequences of these actions are (Schegloff, 1995). The idea that naturally occurring interaction is structurally organized is manifested in a study of general rules and practices of interaction which are assumed to be shared by all competent members of society. Key conversation-analytic discoveries deal with turn-taking (Sacks, Schegloff, & Jefferson, 1974), sequence organization (Schegloff, 2007), repair (Schegloff, Jefferson & Sacks, 1977), and the overall structure of conversational encounters (Schegloff, & Sacks, 1973). Conversation analysis considers talk as central to intersubjectivity, assuming that the processes by which it is constructed become visible in and through participants' displayed understanding of prior talk. For example, by uttering a turn that is hearable as an answer, a speaker demonstrates that he has interpreted the prior turn as a question.

Conversation analysis seeks to investigate data on its own premises. The idea of "unmotivated looking" (e.g., Hoey & Kendrick, 2017) refers to the researcher approaching the data without hypotheses and categories created beforehand, while the phenomena worth studying are assumed to become visible to the researcher through inductive data investigation. The researcher proceeds case by case, attempting to find recurring patterns in these cases. Cases that appear to deviate from the established patterns are analyzed thoroughly as "deviant cases" and their analysis is incorporated in the understanding of those normative patterns that participants usually orient to (Clayman & Maynard, 1995, cf. Liddicoat, 2011; ten Have, 2007). There is only one reality that all competent members of society orient to, and conversation analysis is about unraveling the features of this reality. Since the 1990s, however, with the rise of conversation-analytic studies of institutional interaction (Drew & Heritage, 1992), various asymmetries have been brought to the fore as an inherent part of interaction (Linell & Luckmann, 1991). More specifically, such asymmetries may have to do with *language*, *know-how*, *knowledge*, and *participation* (e.g., Heritage, 1997; Linell, 1998). Such asymmetries also invoke the question about the existence of alternative realities for participants with different degrees of interactional competence.

Asymmetries of language arise in situations in which one or more participants have restricted language skills, for example, due to neurological or developmental problems or because the spoken language is not the person's first language. If a participant has difficulties expressing him or herself, others will need to move the conversation forward, for example, by posing questions or making interpretations of the participant's contributions (Linell, 1998). Previous conversation-analytic research on linguistically asymmetric interaction has sought to describe such difficulties in various clinical populations, such as aphasia (e.g., Goodwin, 2003; Laakso, 1997), autism spectrum disorder (Maynard, 2005; Stevanovic et al., 2017), and dementia (Guendouzi & Müller, 2005; Lindholm, 2015; Mikesell, 2009). In mental health contexts, asymmetries of language are often connected to asymmetries of knowledge (see below). In cases of psychosis, it has been suggested that communication problems between doctors and patients have been due both to the fact that the doctors do not have access to the patients' anomalous experiences and that the patients struggle to describe these experiences (McCabe & Healey, 2018; McCabe, Heath, Burns, & Priebe, 2002).

Asymmetries of know-how refer to the participants' different levels of practical skill. In institutional contexts, such skills may have to do with knowledge about the established practices of the institution. While the institutional encounters are usually routine for the institutional representatives, they are typically unique for the laypersons, who do not have access to the professional's agenda. Routine institutional contingencies can therefore cause confusion for the participants not familiar with the routines. In medicine, the asymmetries of know-how have been shown to cause specific difficulties for vulnerable groups such as children and persons with mental health problems, which has given rise to a movement to promote client-centeredness and shared decision-making practices (Heritage, 2013a). The asymmetries of know-how have also been observed in other types of institutional talk, such as emergency service calls (Whalen, Zimmerman, & Whalen, 1988), courtroom interaction (Drew, 1992), social service encounters (Heritage & Sefi, 1992), and counseling (Peräkylä, 1995). Asymmetries of know-how can also be connected to asymmetries of language. In institutional interactions, it is typically the professional who is responsible for compiling a written report on the basis of the encounter (Agar, 1985). Sometimes, however, a layperson can be put in charge of the written documentation. In such instances, the asymmetries of language and know-how nonetheless tend to trump the predetermined responsibilities: it is usually the person with the greatest linguistic competence who ends up creating the final formulations accepted by the institution (Stevanovic et al., forthcoming).

Asymmetries of knowledge, also known as epistemic asymmetries, involve differences in participants' access to information and rights to articulate that information. In institutional interactions, epistemic asymmetries are typically connected to the professional and lay roles. Usually, the professional has the right to institutionally relevant knowledge, whereas lay knowledge is often hidden and can be easily ignored. In other words, even if the layperson might have institutionally relevant information, he or she may not have the epistemic right to articulate their knowledge (Heritage, 1997). This is often the case in psychiatry where patients lifeworld explanations for their problems are differentiated from the diagnostic explanations provided by clinicians (Weiste, Peräkylä, Valkeapää, Savander, & Hintikka, 2018). A typical example of such asymmetry is also the encounter between a doctor and a patient when the participants orient to having radically differentiated access to medical knowledge (Heritage, 2013b; Lindström & Weatherall, 2015). Thus, patients who use medical terminology or assert medical diagnoses to doctors typically choose to signal tentativeness or hesitation by linguistic markers or certain turn design (Heritage & Raymond, 2005; Heritage & Robinson, 2006). In contrast, psychotherapy involve specific kind of knowledge asymmetry as the talk mainly concerns the client's experiences which are unavailable to the therapist as such. Thus, the clients hold therapists accountable to signal tentativeness in their talk while describing the client's inner experiences (Weiste, Voutilainen, & Peräkylä, 2016).

Finally, *asymmetries of participation* can arise in any situation, but they are particularly common in institutional encounters in which the participants have different and complementary roles connected to certain rights and duties. Typically, these rights and duties involve the institutional representative being responsible for the institutional activities, whereas the layperson is supposed to act in a manner expected by the institution. Asymmetries of participation then become visible in the turn-taking patterns: the professional usually has the right and duty to produce initiatives, whereas the role of the layperson may be restricted to responding to these initiatives. This type of asymmetry, categorized by Robinson (2001) as the "asymmetry of the initiative," has been a topic of a wide range of conversation-analytic studies, focusing on questions and responses in medical interactions (e.g., Boyd & Heritage, 2006; Heritage & Robinson, 2006; Ruusuvuori, 2000). In this volume, we will consider such asymmetries in the context of decision-making sequences, where the distribution of initiatives and responses has immediate consequences for the laypersons' ability and opportunity to influence issues that affect their own lives, health, and welfare.

In joint decision-making interaction, all the different types of asymmetries discussed above become relevant. Asymmetries of language may result in the linguistically most competent participants taking on responsibility to forward the decision-making interactions, which may lead to unilateral decision-making. Asymmetries of know-how may lead to the inequality of the relative weight between the participants' interactional contributions, the more skilled participant being able to summarize and formulate the central turning points in the interaction and thereby control the unfolding of decision-making interaction on a meta-level. Similarly, asymmetries of knowledge have direct consequences for the interactional import of the participants' utterances, the utterances of an expert being more likely to influence the decision-making outcome than the ones spoken by a nonexpert. Finally, asymmetries of participation directly compromise the jointness of the outcome of decision-making interaction: the decision.

Conversation-Analytic Approach to Joint Decision-Making

During the past few decades, several lines of conversation-analytic research on joint decision-making have emerged. These bodies of research share the view of joint decision-making as a process that is both structured and dynamic. Decision-making is essentially action-oriented, involving "a commitment to future action" (Huisman, 2001, p. 70). How participants coordinately end up reaching that commitment, and how they position themselves at different points of the decision-making process, are questions at the heart of this research field.

There has been a long tradition of conversation-analytic studies on negotiations in conflictual contexts, in which disagreements are largely expected (Firth, 1995). In an early work, Bilmes (1981) studied decision-making in a task-based discussion in the Federal Trade Commission, focusing particularly on the participants' ways of demarcating and adjusting individual opinions in order to reach a socially acceptable outcome. In a similar vein, Bilmes (1995) demonstrated how agreement emerges as the parties closely monitor and contingently respond to each other's positions as those positions unfold. In contrast, in her study on a formal union-management negotiation event, Walker (1995) pointed to the participants' preexisting conflictual positions being reflected in their formulations consistently making tendentious interpretations of prior talk. Only formulations arising during the "concessionary phases" of the negotiation process implied a resolution, "providing an opportunity for the two sides to reach agreement" (p. 103).

Boden (1994, 1995) raised the study of meetings to the forefront of conversation analysis, revealing new aspects of decision-making in organizational environments. She investigated internal meetings held in a hospital, a TV station, and a department within a university administration, noting especially the persuasive function of "reformulations." She showed that proposers constantly monitor the reception of their proposals and within a fraction of a second, reformulate it in an attempt to arrive at a mutually acceptable decision. Huisman (2001), then again, criticized the notion of decisions as concrete, manifest "things" that participants can take away with them from a meeting. Instead, she emphasized the character of organizational decision-making as an incremental activity. While participants move their agendas forward step-by-step, it is not always obvious whether and when a decision has been established. Huisman argued that the emergence of decisions depends on the communicative norms of the given group—what, in each context, counts as a decision.

Conversation-analytic research on organizational decision-making has also drawn attention to meetings as a site for determining and negotiating social relationships including one's status and ranking. Clifton (2009) described differentiated practices used by superordinate and subordinate persons to achieve influence in decision-making in a business meeting: while a superordinate may use formulations in reliance of category-bound resources of the chairperson, a subordinate person needs to allow the chair to take ownership of decision-making in order to be able to achieve influence. Clifton (2009) also demonstrated how a superordinate could close an episode of talk and retrospectively orient to it as a decision. In a similar vein, Asmuss and Oshima (2012) showed how participants in a meeting oriented both to the acceptance or rejection of proposals, and to the participants' differentiated rights to make a proposal and to accept or reject it. This multilayeredness of proposals became apparent in the participants being able to accept a proposal while at the same time disagreeing with the decision-making rights, and vice versa. More generally, the idea of participants orienting to their respective rights to propose and decide has been captured by the notion of *deontic authority* (Bochenski, 1974; Stevanovic & Peräkylä, 2012) or *deontic rights* (Stevanovic, 2013, 2018).

There is also a body of conversation-analytic studies on joint decision-making in multiprofessional teamwork. In their study of teams of student designers, Campbell, Roth, and Jornet (2019) described team decision-making as involving a general three-phase structure. The structure involves the design options first emerging as the team members respond to the unfolding situation, which is followed by the team members creating preferences toward the emerged options and, finally, selecting from among the options. Multiprofessional teamwork is often motivated by the idea of different participants' possessing specialist knowledge and expertise in distinct fields. Thus, in addition to the participants' respective deontic rights discussed above, studies on multiprofessional teamwork make particularly relevant the notion of *epistemic authority* (Bochenski, 1974; Heritage & Raymond, 2005) or *epistemic rights* (Raymond & Heritage, 2006). In focusing on the "knowledge claims that interactants assert, contest and defend in and through turns at talk and sequences of interaction" (Heritage, 2013b, p. 370), conversation-analytic research on epistemics has emphasized the need to consider "the in situ interactional characteristics of the exchange of information and the recognition of knowledgeable utterances within team-based contexts" (Housley, 2000, p. 104). In this vein, Housley (2000) examined how utterances produced in a multiprofessional team meeting were interactionally recognized as displays of authoritative knowledge. He demonstrated how knowledge, as an emergent and occasioned product of team interaction, depends on claims of validity, which in turn may be backed up by the use of professional membership categories.

Besides various institutional contexts, everyday family interactions are an important locus of joint decision-making. LeBlanc (2018) examined practices of "doing" family relationships, pointing to the importance of planning future shared events as an indication of expectations of continued being together. De Stefani (2013) examined couples shopping in a supermarket, describing how they made the "committed" dimension of their relationship publicly visible in and through joint shopping decisions. De Stefani (2014) also identified three phases in how shoppers systematically and methodically establish joint orientation toward an object. These phases involve one person introducing a new referent, the other person acknowledging it and displaying a change of orientation, and, finally, one of them commenting, assessing, or asking about it or issuing a directive. In this way, decisions regarding an object's "purchasability" come across as collaborative achievements.

While most conversation-analytic studies of joint decision-making practices have addressed the practices and normative orientations of participants who may be classified as fully competent members of society, a few exceptions are worth noting, however. Krummheuer (2020) investigated shopping decisions done by a person with acquired brain injury in collaboration with her caregiver. While the caregiver's primary task was to provide instrumental assistance that is oriented toward the client's physical impairment (e.g., taking objects down from the shelf), Krummheuer showed that the caregiver also oriented to the client's ability to make the "right" choice, thus undermining the client's moral agency. Similar orientations to the lack of the clients' deontic rights in relation to their own preferences have also been observed in the context of dementia care (Lindholm & Stevanovic, 2020/in press). As for the impact of mental illness on joint decision-making practices, McCabe and Lavelle (2012) conducted a conversation-analytic study on joint decision-making in an experimental setting. Their findings pointed to some schizophrenia-related atypicalities in the management of turn exchanges: failing to take the opportunity to speak when offered one and beginning to speak from the role of an unaddressed recipient.

In sum, there is a rich body of conversation-analytic studies on the structural features of joint decision-making. According to these studies, the usual starting point of joint decision-making is a *proposal* for a future action or event, or—as Huisman (2001) put it—a "formulation of a state of affairs that is of current interest" (p. 72). However, proposals themselves may come in a variety of forms—"as suggestions, requests, inquiries, 'musings' and so on" (Francis, 1995, p. 41), which means that in order to launch joint decision-making, they must be recognized as proposals. Francis (1995) has stressed the importance of shared responsibilities and tasks in this respect: in his view, "only by virtue of such common concerns is an action recognisable as a proposal in the first place" (p. 56). A joint decision may then be defined as one possible outcome of the participants' subsequent treatment of turns that have been recognized as proposals. An early version of this idea is presented in an early study on plea bargaining by Maynard (1984), who described what he termed "the bargaining sequence." This sequence consists of a proposal or report of a preference and the other party's alignment or misalignment with the first turn, the aligning response leading to a decision. Similarly, Houtkoop (1987) pointed to agreement as dependent on the recipients' subsequent treatment of proposals. In line with the classical findings on preference structure (Davidson, 1984; Pomerantz, 1984), Houtkoop demonstrated that rejection is often delayed, whereas acceptance is commonly done straight away. Importantly, however, Houtkoop (1987) also showed that responses to proposals for immediate vs. remote actions—that is, actions to be carried out now vs. later—take different forms. Whereas immediate proposals lead to a three-part sequence (proposal, acceptance, and acknowledgment), remote proposals usually have a five-part structure (proposal, acceptance, request for confirmation, confirmation, and acknowledgment). Drawing on these insights, Stevanovic (2012) has further specified the characteristics of joint decision-making sequences following remote proposals. She suggested that joint decisions emerge when the recipients' accepting responses to proposals contain three components: a claim of understanding what the proposal is about (*access*), an indication that the proposed plan is feasible (*agreement*), and a demonstration of willingness to treat the plan as binding (*commitment*). If the recipient abandons the sequence before providing all these components, the proposal is de facto rejected, without the recipient needing to produce an explicit rejection of the proposal.

Joint decision-making is a social phenomenon in its own right, defined as a "set of actions, operations, and dynamic factors that start with the identification of a stimulus for action and end with a commitment to action" (Campbell et al., 2019, p. 3). In this volume, we want to advance understanding of this social phenomenon. We maintain that the social world with its entire web of social relations is constructed, negotiated, and played out in the turn-by-turn unfolding of joint decision-making interaction, which happens when participants respond to each other's proposals or silently ignore them. From this perspective, joint decision-making sequences are a site of continuous power struggle—one in which the sequential trajectories of turns at talk, not only confirm or challenge participants' understandings of self (Stevanovic & Peräkylä, 2012; Stevanovic & Svennevig, 2015) but also have tangible consequences for the participants involved.

Joint Decision-Making in Clinical Encounters

Within the field of CA, joint decision-making has been much examined in medical settings. These studies have described how treatment decisions are negotiated, delivered, justified, accepted, or rejected in the contexts of primary and secondary care, including psychiatry (Gill & Roberts, 2014). In this section, we will outline some of the findings from this area of study, focusing especially on decision-making in mental health care.

An important topic in this field of research is the delivery of treatment recommendations. Stivers and colleagues (2018) found that in primary care treatment, recommendations are typically delivered through pronouncements, suggestions, proposals, and offers. The same recommendation forms are also used in psychiatric outpatient clinics (Thompson & McCabe, 2018). The choice of the recommendation form is important as it shapes the clinician's epistemic and deontic authority relative to the client. In pronouncements, clinicians exploit their epistemic and deontic authority over the client (Stivers et al., 2018). In suggestions, clinicians maintain epistemic authority over the recommendation but refrain from exerting deontic authority. In proposals, clinicians not only share their deontic rights with the clients but may also reduce their epistemic authority by presenting their treatment recommendations as speculative. In offers, clinicians relinquish their deontic authority and imply client's agency as the driving force behind the recommendation. (Stivers et al., 2018). In a similar vein, Toerien, Shaw, and Reuber (2013) described the practice of option-listing as a way for the clinicians work to abdicate some of their medical authority and create more space for the client to participate (Toerien et al., 2013). In the context of psychiatry, it has also been noticed that clinicians pull back from their authoritarian position and support client participation (e.g., Angell & Bolden, 2015; Kushida & Yamakawa, 2015; McCabe et al., 2002). Such "pulling back" has been typically achieved by delivering treatment recommendations as proposals (Thompson & McCabe, 2018). Moreover, using those proposal forms that shared some surface-level features of open proposals, while yet constraining the clients' response options to be either in favor or against one already set-out action plan (so called "quasi open" proposals), has been shown to best encourage client responsiveness in the context of mental health rehabilitation (Stevanovic, Valkeapää, Weiste, & Lindholm, 2020/in press).

The management of medical authority during clinical encounters has been described with reference to the decision-making communication being "unilateral" vs. "bilateral." For instance, Collins, Drew, Watt, and Entwistle (2005) studied decision-making in primary care and specialist oncology encounters, describing how unilateral decisions emerged when clinicians' suggestions, recommendations, or conclusions made relevant the client's acceptance of the decision, rather than their further contribution to it. In contrast, bilateral decisions emerged when more elaborated client contributions were invited. Bilateral decision-making pattern involved specific elicitation of client's views and experiences, which were then further integrated into clinicians' medical options (Collins et al., 2005). Ijäs-Kallio, Ruusuvuori, and Peräkylä (2011) studied how patients respond to unilateral decisions in Finnish primary care consultations, finding that clients could challenge such decisions by extended responses that invited negotiation on the decision.

Personal pronouns are an important resource in marking a decision as uni- or bilateral. In Thompson and McCabe's study (2018) on British psychiatric outpatient encounters, the clinicians used "we"-formulated proposals to implicate shared decisional accountability and partnership between the clinician and the client. Also, Kushida and Yamakawa (2015) showed that in Japanese outpatient consultations, psychiatrists used the inclusive "we"-form in their proposals, when the sequential environment was ready for making an actual treatment decision. However, "we" can also be used to invoke the psychiatrist's medical authority. When a client resists a medication decision, the "institutional we" may be used to invoke a multidisciplinary treatment team to side with the psychiatrist (Angell & Bolden, 2016).

CA research across different medical settings has pointed to a common pattern that involves both clinicians and clients orienting to treatment recommendations as normatively requiring client acceptance (Stivers, 2005). Through acceptance, withholding of acceptance, or active resistance, clients can negotiate a treatment outcome that is in line with their preferences (Stivers, 2005). Passive resistance has been shown to be the most common manifestation of client resistance. By analyzing parental resistance to GPs' treatment recommendations, Stivers (2006) described passive resistance as involving an absence of the expected client response to the treatment recommendation made by the clinician. Such absence may be achieved either through a nonresponse or by moving the conversation away from the recommendation. Then again, active resistence may involve the clients either disagreeing with the clinician's recommendations or discouraging anticipated recommendations even before the clinicians have made them (Gill, Pomerantz, & Denvir, 2010; Stivers, 2006).

In the context of psychiatry, the overt resistance of the client has been noted often to be in response to proposals and offers which characterized *less* psychiatrist (and more client) responsibility (Thompson & McCabe, 2018). Also, Angell and Bolden's (2015) study indicates that clinicians' client-centric accounts for or against changes in medication may be more vulnerable to client resistance than authority-oriented accounts. They suggest that stepping on the client's epistemic domain by addressing their experiences may invoke client resistance (Angell & Bolden, 2015). Dealing with client resistance can sometimes also lead to an escalating cycle of pressure and disagreement. Quirk, Chapin, Lelliott, and Seale (2012) studied instances of explicit disagreement, when a psychiatrist responded to client resistance by pressuring the client to agree, in which case the decision-making situation was difficult to bring to a close without either the client or the psychiatrist losing face.

Client resistance is often presented as a problem that professionals must overcome to be able to secure a clinically desirable outcome (see e.g., Pilnick & Coleman, 2003). It is therefore interesting to note that client resistance has also been considered to be a significant resource of client participation (Barton et al., 2016). According to this argument, it is in and through their resistance to clinicians' treatment recommendations that clients can work to negotiate and collaboratively co-construct what counts as an acceptable decision (Koenig, 2011). This paradoxical role of client resistance as both a "hinderer" and "enabler" of participation is one of the central threads in the volume, which characterizes particularly its first empirical part.

Dimensions of Joint Decision-Making Sequences

This volume addresses several gaps in the conversation-analytic literature on joint decision-making in mental health care contexts. First, while most previous research has concentrated on doctor–patient interaction, this volume includes a broader range of encounters with individuals with mental health problems, including psychotherapy, occupational therapy, and community rehabilitation. Second, little is known about decision-making in mental health encounters involving more than two participants. By studying triadic and multiparty settings, this volume offers new insights into how the number of participants affects decision-making trajectories. Third, and finally, this volume involves data from a broad set of different clinical groups. This broad dataset helps to distinguish between those features that characterize all interactions and those that can be best accounted for with reference to the specific challenges that persons with mental illnesses face in joint decision-making.

As the chapters in this volume demonstrate, joint decision-making is a complex phenomenon. This complexity may be clarified with reference to a range of dimensions: (1) context, (2) content, (3) action design, and (4) interactional patterns. Below, we introduce these dimensions in more detail, hoping that they will aid future research on joint decision-making.

Context

Joint decision-making is always embedded in some external or structural configurations that both enable and constrain the activity, while these can be of various extents, scales, and degrees of public visibility. However, their essential feature is that they can be oriented to as "given" at each moment of interaction, even if they are subject to constant change.

Constellation of the encounter. The number of participants in the encounter has been shown to have a significant impact on structures of social interaction, such as on the organization of turn-taking and participation (e.g., Schegloff, 1995). The constellation of the encounter also plays a role in the formation of decisions (see e.g., Kangasharju, 2002). This volume features decision-making in both two-party interactions (Chapters 4, 5, 7, and 10) and multiparty interactions (Chapters 2, 3, 6, 8, 9, 11, and 12), pointing to the specific challenges that client resistance may generate in multiparty interactions.

Participants' mutual relationships. The question of who the participants are to each other is a central aspect of the context of joint decision-making. The participants' relationships may be anchored in their predefined institutional roles but other factors, such as the participants' common personal history and the sociocultural expectations that guide the formation of social relations, also play a role in this regard. This volume highlights the epistemic and deontic facets of participants' mutual relationships, analyzing how clients typically avoid challenging their authority, even when resisting doctors' treatment recommendations (Chapter 5). Another relationship facet considered in the volume is the degree of familiarity between the participants (Chapter 7).

Assumptions of competence. While the idea about general rules and practices of interaction as shared by all competent members of society offers a fruitful basis for conversation-analytic research, assumptions of competence must be relaxed in the types of asymmetric data studied in this volume. As soon as we get the sense that one interactional participant orients to a lack of competence in another and therefore modifies their trajectory of action from what it might have otherwise been, we must consider the possibility of alternative interactional realities. From this perspective, the analysis of joint decision-making sequences depends crucially on how capable participants may be assumed to be in expressing their disagreement with what is about to emerge as a decision (Chapter 12; see also Bilmes, 1995).

Implicit goals and agendas. Participants' implicit goals and agendas are a significant part of the "invisible" context of joint decision-making. In the studies in this volume, one such goal involves professionals acting in accordance with client-centered ideology. Another goal that many professionals seem to have involves socializing clients into the practices of joint decision-making. Indirect indices of such agendas may be seen in professionals engaging in prospective and retrospective framing of decision-making episodes explicitly as consensus-based and in what may be called "vicarious participation" (Chapter 12). However, there are also contexts in which no explicit decisions are sought for, but the "mere" construction of joint meaning is treated as enough (Chapter 11).

Task expectations. Finally, the participants' sociocultural expectations related to the task at hand constitute a central aspect of the context for any joint decision-making interaction. For example, participants may orient to preexisting conflictual positions between them and to a need to defend their views and refrain from premature displays of agreement (Walker, 1995). While some studies reported in this volume exhibit similar conflictual positions (Chapters 3 and 7), in most studies the participants seem to orient to relatively consensual positions. Decision-making tasks may also be surrounded by different expectations of responsibility, often the professionals being more in charge of the emergence of the decisions than the clients (Chapter 2).

Content

Sequences of joint decision-making further differ regarding their content. In the present volume, the decisions discussed are generally about clients' medications (Chapters 3, 5, and 7), behavioral changes (Chapter 4), activity performances (Chapter 11), as well as working procedures and discussion topics of a rehabilitation group (Chapters 2, 6, 8, 10, and 12). The decisions also vary regarding their immediateness and consequences.

Immediateness of decisions. Decisions concern action to be realized immediately or in the future (Houtkoop, 1987). For instance, occupational therapists invite client proposals to decide how to solve problems related to their shared activity performance, and the decision is executed immediately when the participants continue the activity at hand (Chapter 9). In most studies in this volume, however, the decisions concern clients' future actions, such as behavioral changes (Chapter 4) or medication intake (Chapters 3, 5, and 7).

Consequences of decisions. Joint decision-making can encompass both high and low-stakes decisions. In this volume, the high-stakes decisions are commonly treatment decisions (Chapters 3, 5, and 7), whereas low-stakes decisions concern small-scale everyday activities (Chapters 2, 4, 6, 8, 10, and 12). Joint decision-making sequences also vary regarding the distribution of consequences of the decision for different participants.

Action Design

The decision-making sequences analyzed also make differentiated use of basic turn- and action-design features, which have been abundantly discussed in conversation-analytic literature on action ascription and formation (for an overview, see Levinson, 2013).

Linguistic resources. Personal pronouns comprise one significant linguistic resource to manage participation and social inclusion and is therefore also relevant to joint decision-making. Interaction involving more than two participants involves an increased demand for managing recipiency, which manifests itself as changes in the turn-taking organization compared to the patterns of two-party conversations. Whereas referring to a person with a second-person reference is unproblematic in dyads, a setting involving multiple recipients may call for a more frequent use of names and noun phrases to identify the recipient (Schegloff, 1996). In this volume, Chapter 9 shows how the professional uses second-person plural forms ("we") to address recipients in proposal sequences. Pronouns are also used to indicate whether participants orient toward others or themselves in their turns. The analysis in Chapter 6 demonstrates how the use of second-person singular pronouns display other-orientation, whereas first-person plural pronouns are used to refer to the whole group including the speaker.

Embodied resources. Except for linguistic resources, embodied resources are used to refer to a recipient and to provoke responses (Goodwin, 1981; Lerner, 1996). This is exemplified in Chapter 9, which reports on an analysis of how pronoun use is combined with gaze to select the next speaker. The regulatory function of gaze in interaction is well-known in the conversation-analytic literature. For example, Stivers and Rossano (2010) discuss speaker gaze to recipient as one of the main means of pursuing a response.

Material objects. The material objects with which participants are currently engaged may be crucial for joint decision-making. For instance, Fazulo and Monzoni (2009) have shown that negative assessments of objects with which participants are currently engaged, can function as proposals. Objects can also be used for inviting proposals from others. Chapter 10 illustrates how occupational therapists elicit client proposals by publicly noticing physical objects in the therapy room. Also, the act of writing is central to decision-making (e.g., Nissi, 2015). Chapter 8 shows how writing and editing previously written texts can serve joint decision-making by transforming vague ideas into potentially serious proposals.

Interactional Patterns

Joint decision-making sequences also exhibit patterns that emerge solely between the participants as a result of their intertwined actions.

(A)symmetry of participation. Joint decision-making sequences demonstrate variation in terms of participation dynamics. Most evidently, both the amount of talk and the number of strong versus weak interactional moves allocated to participants vary, which may be particularly common in institutional settings with specific role-based expectations (Drew & Heritage, 1992). Chapter 2 features instances of support workers pursuing a response in situations in which the clients do not respond to the support workers' initiatives. These instances exemplify that the support workers have the right and obligation to take the agenda forward by producing strong initiative moves, whereas the clients' rights may be restricted to responding to these initiatives.

Party formation. Sequences of joint decision-making are further diverse in the degree to which they involve the formation of subgroups or oppositional alliances (Kangasharju, 1996, 2002). Chapter 3 exemplifies how clinicians and parents may create alliances in discussions about medical treatment at the psychiatrist's practice, whereas children, even though invited to share their perspective, are excluded from the ultimate decision about the treatment. Chapter 9, then again, demonstrates how support workers temporarily categorize clients as an outgroup separate from the support workers by addressing them with second-person plural forms. Paradoxically, this seems to function as an effective manner to encourage clients' participation in group interaction.

Pace of decision-making. Sometimes joint decisions emerge quickly, sometimes this takes much time. As outlined in Chapter 6, the pace typically differs between two-party and multiparty conversations. In dyads, the decision-making can unproblematically move swiftly toward a decision, but in multiparty interaction the outcome of the proposal needs to be constructed as a joint decision to which all participants are committed. The pace of the decision-making may therefore need to be slowed down in order to enable everybody to contribute to the decision before the sequence ends. Chapter 10 exemplifies how the occupational therapist, instead of solving a problem herself, gives room to the client to propose a solution. The slower pace provides the client with an opportunity to decide how to proceed.

Influence on the agenda. Joint decision-making sequences also vary with respect to the degree of influence that a person's interactional contribution (e.g., a proposal) exerts on the agenda of the encounter. Interestingly, such influence seems to be independent of the matter of acceptance versus rejection of the content of that contribution. For example, in the group conversations in Chapter 6, a professional accepts the client's proposal immediately, thereby providing the group with very limited room to elaborate on the client's views. The situation is the opposite in Chapter 7, in which a psychiatrist rejects a client's request for a change of medication, while yet allowing them to have a substantial impact on the agenda of the encounter.

Publicity in the emergence of the final decision. The decision-making sequences analyzed in this volume also vary in how clear it is whether and when a decision gets established. Occasionally, participants explicitly display their orientation to the principles of decision-making. An illustration is provided in Chapter 8, which illustrates how participants can treat writing down a suggestion as an indication of establishing a decision. The established decisions can nevertheless be more or less binding.

(Mis)alignment concerning the ownership of decisions. Joint decision-making sequences are a locus of implicit negotiation of agency, power, and deontic authority (Stevanovic, 2018). From this perspective, proposals and their accepting responses can often exhibit subtle patterns of misalignment. The participants could agree fully with the content of a decision but still disagree with the "ownership" of the decision. Thus, analogous to findings about participants using argumentation in contexts where everyone agrees (Mundwiler & Kreuz, 2018), a decision may be accompanied with elaborations that draw attention to the role of the speaker as somebody who has the final say in the matter. While such claims of ownership may be accepted by others, they can sometimes be followed by implicit challenges and negotiations (Clifton, 2009). However, as suggested in Chapter 6, it is possible that "high-involvement communication" (Tannen, 2005) works to neutralize such competition, as the collaborative mode of thinking starts to dominate over individualistic concerns.

Meta-management of jointness. Finally, the jointness of decision-making sequences can be constructed through both words and actions. Thus, participants can engage in meta-talk describing the decision-making as joint and shared, and they can perform actions indicating an orientation to shared decisions. Chapters 7 and 12 demonstrate that these two manners of constructing jointness are not always in line with each other. Chapter 7 exemplifies how psychiatrists, although rejecting clients' requests, may present their decisions as bilateral and being in line with what the clients had requested. By using collective reference forms and acknowledging the client's epistemic authority over his bodily experiences, the psychiatrist validates the client's involvement in treatment decisions. Chapter 12 provides a detailed illustration of how words and actions are not necessarily in line with each other. In this chapter, the support worker makes explicit references to the ideal of consensus-based decision-making. The decision-making sequences are both prospectively and retrospectively framed as matching with the ideals of consensus-based decision-making, but simultaneously, the support worker may direct the conversation so that only specific types of responses are promoted. Consensus-based decision-making is thus demonstrated to be a difficult ideal to realize and it is held together with much meta-management of jointness.

Volume Overview

The remainder of this volume consists of 10 empirical chapters, divided into three sections dealing with different aspects of joint decision-making in interactions between professionals and clients with mental illness. The three sections are entitled: *Client Silence and Resistance*, *Professionals Responding to Clients*, and *Discourse and Ideology*.

Client Silence and Resistance

The first empirical section seeks to address head-on the challenges faced by many professionals in the context of mental health—that is, the problems in the realization of the ideal of shared decision-making in practice (see Beitinger, Kissling, & Hamann, 2014; De las Cuevas, Rivero-Santana, Perestelo-Pérez, Pérez-Ramos, & Serrano-Aguilar, 2012; Elstad & Eide, 2009; Ernst & Paulus, 2005; Hickey & Kipping, 1998; Larquet et al., 2010; Stovell, Morrison, Panayiotou, & Hutton, 2016). The three chapters in the section provide detailed analyses of the professionals' attempts to promote client participation taking place in the face of client silence. The analyses of these chapters also address client resistance and the professional's ways of dealing with it as multifaceted phenomena by which the recognition of clients as legitimate decision-makers is specifically at stake.

The section starts with Melisa Stevanovic, Taina Valkeapää, Elina Weiste, and Camilla Lindholm analyzing support workers' practices to facilitate participation in mental health rehabilitation group meetings at a Clubhouse community. The support workers are shown to treat clients' turns retrospectively as proposals, remind clients about their access to the proposed idea and pursue their agreement or commitment to it. While these practices are fundamentally cooperative, they are dilemmatic in that they deprive the clients the opportunity to use silence as a resource of implicit resistance.

In Chapter 3, Lisa Mikesell, Alethia Marti, Jennifer R. Guzmán, Michael McCreary, and Bonnie Zima examine treatment decisions of children diagnosed with attention deficit hyperactivity disorder (ADHD), who seem to adopt a passive role in participating in decision-making about their medication. The authors show how the clinicians' attempts to invite children's participation commonly occur only after the parent has already accepted a specific treatment. While the clinicians thus recognize children's role in the decision-making process, they nonetheless attend to the primary authority of the parents to make decisions for their children.

In Chapter 4, Katie Ekberg and Amanda LeCouteur analyze how cognitive behavioral therapists invite clients to share responsibility for decision-making about therapy goals on behavior change. The therapists' information-soliciting questions are shown to position the clients as knowledgeable about and as having the right to suggest how to change their own behavior. In contrast, the therapists' own proposals for behavior change imply therapists' superior right to tell clients what to do. Clients are shown to systematically resist these therapists' proposals, invoking their own epistemic and deontic authority over the situation.

Chapter 5, authored by Shuya Kushida and Yuriko Yamakawa, shows how patient resistance to psychiatrists' treatment recommendations can embody patients' agency and enhance their participation in decision-making. As ways of resisting the recommendation, the patients may query the effectiveness of the recommended treatment or reveal their experiences of the negative effects of the treatment. By formulating the obstacles for accepting the recommendation as falling within their own epistemic territory, the patients can resist the treatment recommendations without explicitly challenging the psychiatrists' authority.

Professionals Responding to Clients

While discussion in the first section is about how clinicians encourage, recognize, and maintain the legitimacy of client participation in the face of client silence and resistance, in the second section, in contrast, is a consideration of clients as initiators of joint decision-making activities and professionals as for their ways of responding to clients. The chapters in this section explore the professionals' balancing between recognizing the clients' status as legitimate actors in joint decision-making while also taking care of the accomplishment of those institutional tasks for which the professionals alone are responsible.

In Chapter 6, Stevanovic and colleagues address two dilemmas that professionals may face when responding to the clients' proposals in group meetings. The first dilemma has to do with the professionals needing to provide individual clients recognition for their proposals, while enthusiastic approval of these proposals may discourage further group participation. The second dilemma involves the professionals seeking to focus on the clients as the originators of their proposal, which may lead to constructing an individual client alone as accountable for his or her proposal and indicate a lack of its relevance for the whole group.

Chapter 7, authored by Galina B. Bolden, Alexa Hepburn, and Beth Angell, explores medication decisions in psychiatric community outpatient clinics. Focusing on clients' requests for medication changes and psychiatrists' responses to these requests, it is demonstrated that psychiatrists make an active effort to validate client participation—both in cases when the clients' requests are handled seriously and when they are dismissed without investigation. The psychiatrists accomplish this through the interactional practices of asking questions to assess grounds for the clients' requests, agreeing with their assessments, and pursuing their acceptance of treatment decisions.

In Chapter 8, Lindholm and colleagues discuss how writing may be invoked as a resource by professionals to incorporate clients' insights into decision-making processes. By studying rehabilitation group meetings at the Clubhouse, the chapter shows how the activity of editing previously written texts allows for collective access to the ideas "in the air." Furthermore, the act of writing may transform vague and nonspecific ideas into proposals to be potentially taken seriously later on. Moreover, a reference to a written piece of text may be used as a way to end a prolonged decision-making sequence.

Discourse and Ideology

The final section of the volume examines the interplay between ideology and discourse, with the notion of "ideology" representing a set of norms and values that provide the basis for the verbal and embodied conduct at the "discourse" level. The chapters feature analysis of how local resources at the discourse level engage with the ideology. Sometimes such engagement plays out in a paradoxical manner, such as when linguistic features typically associated with values contrary to the underlying ideology are shown to align with it and vice versa.

Chapter 9, by Jenny Paananen and colleagues, focuses on how support workers address clients with second-person plural references during decision-making. According to the Clubhouse ideology, client inclusion involves the reduction of power differences between clients and professionals. However, the analysis reveals that by temporarily distinguishing the clients from themselves, the support workers encourage the client members of the group to share their thoughts. Produced later in the decision-making sequence, the categorization of the clients as an outgroup by the use of second-person plural view elicitors can be interpreted as a demand to agree.

In Chapter 10, Elina Weiste analyzes the making of small-scale decisions during joint activities in occupational therapy sessions at psychiatric outpatient clinics. The therapists are shown to elicit such decision-making moves from the clients by publicly noticing physical objects in the environment and by referring to their problematic features, which allows the clients to exert control over the agenda of the therapeutic sessions. In contrast, when the therapists themselves make small-scale decisions, these are shown to work to help the clients to maintain a clear focus on what to do next.

In Chapter 11, Evrinomy Avdi and Vasileia Lerou discuss the joint creation of new meanings in couple therapy, which may be considered as a specific type of joint decision-making. The authors focus on an ongoing process in psychotherapy which involves clients and therapists creating joint understandings of the clients' difficulties. The negotiations of problem constructions implicate a cause, ascribe responsibility and imply solutions, which are all relevant subprocesses of joint decision-making. The analysis underscores the importance of the therapist's affective responsiveness in facilitating narrative elaboration and emotional expression.

Chapter 12, authored by Taina Valkeapää and co-workers, investigates consensus-based decision-making at the Clubhouse mental health rehabilitation community. The analysis focuses on how decisions are prospectively and retrospectively framed as consensus-based and on how disagreement is managed in interaction. During the decision-making, support workers may also seek to integrate different views and halt the interaction in situations where potential disagreements might go unnoticed. The support workers' practices not only provide clients with local and situational support but also serve as means of socializing them into the social-communicative conventions of the Clubhouse.

References

Agar, M. (1985). Institutional discourse. *Text, 5*(3), 147–168.

Alanko, A., & Hellman, M. (2017). Service users and experts in Finnish mental health care planning: Three phases of expansion and inclusion. *Sosiologia, 54,* 361–376.

Andrews, S. B., Drake, T., Haslett, W., & Munusamy, R. (2010). Developing Web-based online support tools: The Darthmouth decision-support software. *Psychiatric Rehabilitation Journal, 34,* 37–41.

Angell, B., & Bolden, G. B. (2015). Justifying medication decisions in mental health care: Psychiatrists' accounts for treatment recommendations. *Social Science and Medicine, 138,* 44–56.

Angell, B., & Bolden, G. B. (2016). Team work in action: Building grounds for psychiatric medication decisions in assertive community treatment. In M. O'Reilly & J. Lester (Eds.), *The Palgrave handbook of adult mental health* (pp. 371–393). London: Palgrave Macmillan.

Anthony, W. A. (2007). *Toward a vision of recovery: For mental health and psychiatric rehabilitation services*. Boston: Boston University Press.

Asmuss, B., & Oshima, S. (2012). Negotiation of entitlement in proposal sequences. *Discourse Studies, 14*(1), 107–126.

Barton, J., Dew, K., Dowell, A., Sheridan, N., Kenealy, T., Macdonald, L., … Stubbe, M. (2016). Patient resistance as a resource: Candidate obstacles in diabetes consultations. *Sociology of Health & Illness, 38*(7), 1151–1166.

Beitinger, R., Kissling, W., & Hamann, J. (2014). Trends and perspectives of shared decision-making in schizophrenia and related disorders. *Current Opinion in Psychiatry, 27*(3), 222–229.

Bilmes, J. (1981). Proposition and confrontation in a legal discussion. *Semiotica, 34,* 251–275.

Bilmes, J. (1995). Negotiation and compromise: A microanalysis of a discussion in the United States Federal Trade Commission. In A. Firth (Ed.), *The discourse of negotiation: Studies of language in the workplace* (pp. 61–81). Oxford: Pergamon.

Bochenski, J. M. (1974). An analysis of authority. In F. J. Adelman (Ed.), *Authority* (pp. 56–85). The Hague, NL: Martinus Nijhoff.

Boden, D. (1994). *The business of talk: Organizations in action*. Cambridge: Polity Press.

Boden, D. (1995). Agendas and arrangements: Everyday negotiations in meetings. In A. Firth (Ed.), *The discourse of negotiation: Studies of language in the workplace* (pp. 83–99). Oxford: Pergamon.

Boyd, E. H., & Heritage, J. (2006). Taking the patient's medical history. Questioning during comprehensive history taking. In J. Heritage & D. W. Maynard (Eds.), *Communication in medical care: Interaction between primary care physicians and patients* (pp. 151–184). Cambridge: Cambridge University Press.

Campbell, C., Roth, W.-M., & Jornet, A. (2019). Collaborative design decision-making as social process. *European Journal of Engineering Education, 44*(3), 294–311.

Canal, R. (2010). *Social inclusion and participatory democracy: From the conceptual discussion to local action*. UCLG Committee on Social Inclusion, Participatory Democracy and Human Rights. https://www.uclg.org/en/media/news/social-inclusion-and-participatory-democracy-conceptual-discussion-local-action.

Charles, C., Gafni, A., & Whelan, T. (1997). Shared decision-making in the medical encounter: What does it mean? (Or, it takes at least two to tango). *Social Science and Medicine, 44*(5), 681–692.

Clayman, S., & Maynard, D. W. (1995). Ethnomethodology and conversation analysis. In P. ten Have & G. Psathas (Eds.), *Situated order: Studies in the social organization of talk and embodied activities* (pp. 1–30). Washington, DC: University Press of America.

Clifton, J. (2009). Beyond taxonomies of influence: "Doing" influence and making decisions in management team meetings. *Journal of Business Communication, 46*(1), 57–79.

Collins, S., Drew, P., Watt, I., & Entwistle, V. (2005). 'Unilateral' and 'bilateral' practitioner approaches in decision-making about treatment. *Social Science and Medicine, 61*(12), 2611–2627.

Colomy, P., & Brown, J. D. (1996). Goffman and interactional citizenship. *Sociological Perspectives, 39*(3), 371–381.

Crawford, M. J., Rutter, D., Manley, C., Weaver, T., Bhui, K., Fulop, N., & Tyrer, P. (2002). Systematic review of involving patients in the planning and development of health care. *British Medical Journal, 325*(7375), 1263.

Davidson, J. A. (1984). Subsequent versions of invitations, offers, requests, and proposals dealing with potential or actual rejection. In J. M. Atkinson & J. Heritage (Eds.), *Structures of social action: Studies in conversation analysis* (pp. 57–101). Cambridge: Cambridge University Press.

De las Cuevas, C., Rivero-Santana, A., Perestelo-Pérez, L., Pérez-Ramos, J., & Serrano-Aguilar, P. (2012). Attitudes toward concordance in psychiatry: A comparative, cross-sectional study of psychiatric patients and mental health professionals. *BMC Psychiatry, 12*(1), 53.

Department of Health. (2001). *The expert patient: A new approach to chronic disease management in the 21st century*. London: HMSO. http://www.dh.gov.uk.

De Stefani, E. (2013). The collaborative organisation of next actions in a semiotically rich environment: Shopping as a couple. In P. Haddington, L. Mondada, & M. Nevile (Eds.), *Interaction and mobility: Language and the body in motion* (pp. 123–151). Berlin & Boston: De Gruyter.

De Stefani, E. (2014). Establishing joint orientation towards commercial objects in a self-service store: How practices of categorisation matter. In M. Nevile, P. Haddington, T. Heinemann, & M. Rauniomaa (Eds.), *Interacting with objects: Language, materiality and social activity* (pp. 271–294). Amsterdam: Benjamins.

Drew, P. (1992). Contested evidence in courtroom cross-examination: The case of a trial for rape. In P. Drew & J. Heritage (Eds.), *Talk at work: Interaction in institutional settings* (pp. 470–520). Cambridge: Cambridge University Press.

Drew, P., & Heritage, J. (Eds.). (1992). *Talk at work: Language use in institutional and work-place settings*. Cambridge: Cambridge University Press.

Elstad, T. A., & Eide, A. H. (2009). User participation in community mental health services: Exploring the experiences of users and professionals. *Scandinavian Journal of Caring Science, 23*(4), 674–681.

Epstein, R. M., Franks, P., Fiscella, K., Cleveland, G. S., Meldrum, S. C., Kravitz, R. L., & Duberstein, P. R. (2005). Measuring patient-centred communication in patient-physician consultations: Theoretical and practical issues. *Social Science and Medicine, 61*(7), 1516–1528.

Ernst, M., & Paulus, M. P. (2005). Neurobiology of decision making: A selective review from a neurocognitive and clinical perspective. *Biological Psychiatry, 58*(8), 597–604.

Fasulo, A., & Monzoni, C. (2009). Assessing mutable objects: A multimodal analysis. *Research on Language and Social Interaction, 42*(4), 362–376.

Firth, A. (1995). Introduction and overview. In A. Firth (Ed.), *The discourse of negotiation: Studies of language in the workplace* (pp. 3–39). Oxford: Pergamon.

Francis, D. (1995). Negotiation, decision making and formalism: The problem of form and substance in negotiation analysis. In K. Ehlich & J. Wagner (Eds.), *The discourse of business negotiation* (pp. 37–64). Berlin, DE: Mouton de Gruyter.

Gill, V., Pomerantz, A., & Denvir, P. (2010). Pre-emptive resistance: Patients' participation in diagnostic sense-making activities. *Sociology of Health & Illness, 32*(1), 1–20.

Gill, V. T., & Roberts, F. (2014). Conversation analysis in medicine. In J. Sidnell & T. Stivers (Eds.), *The handbook of conversation analysis* (pp. 575–592). Chichester: Wiley Blackwell.

Goffman, E. (1983). Interaction order. *American Sociological Review, 48*(1), 1–17.

Goodwin, C. (1981). *Conversational organization: Interaction between speakers and hearers*. New York, NY: Academic Press.

Goodwin, C. (Ed.). (2003). *Conversation and brain damage*. Oxford: Oxford University Press.

Goossensen, A., Zijlstra, P., & Koopmanschap, M. (2007). Measuring shared decision making processes in psychiatry: Skills versus patient satisfaction. *Patient Education and Counseling, 67*(1), 50–56.

Grob, G. N. (2014). *From asylum to community: Mental health policy in modern America*. Princeton, NJ: Princeton University Press.

Guendouzi, J., & Müller, N. (Eds.). (2005). *Approaches to discourse in dementia*. Mahwah, NJ: Lawrence Erlbaum Associates.

Hänninen, E. (2012). *Choices for recovery: Community-based rehabilitation and the Clubhouse Model as means to mental health reforms*. Helsinki: Finnish Institute for Health and Welfare.

Heritage, J. (1984). *Garfinkel and ethnomethodology*. Cambridge: Polity Press.
Heritage, J. (1997). Conversation analysis and institutional talk: Analysing data. In D. Silverman (Ed.), *Qualitative research: Theory, method and practice* (pp. 161–182). London: Sage.
Heritage, J. (2013a). Language and social institutions: The conversation analytic view. *Journal of Foreign Languages, 36*(4), 2–27.
Heritage, J. (2013b). Epistemics in conversation. In J. Sidnell & T. Stivers (Eds.), *The handbook of conversation analysis* (pp. 370–394). Sussex, UK: Wiley-Blackwell.
Heritage, J., & Raymond, G. (2005). The terms of agreement: Indexing epistemic authority and subordination in talk-in-interaction. *Social Psychology Quarterly, 68*(1), 15–38.
Heritage, J., & Robinson, J. D. (2006). The structure of patients' presenting concerns: Physicians' opening questions. *Health Communication, 19*(2), 89–102.
Heritage, J., & Sefi, S. (1992). Dilemmas of advice: Aspects of the delivery and reception of advice in interactions between health visitors and first-time mothers. In P. Drew & J. Heritage (Eds.), *Talk at work: Language use in institutional and work-place settings* (pp. 359–417). Cambridge: Cambridge University Press.
Hickey, G., & Kipping, C. (1998). Exploring the concept of user involvement in mental health through a participation continuum. *Journal of Clinical Nursing, 7*(1), 83–88.
Hoey, E., & Kendrick, K. (2017). Conversation analysis. In A. M. B. De Groot & P. Hagoort (Eds.), *Research methods in psycholinguistics and the neurobiology of language. A practical guide* (pp. 151–173). Hoboken, NJ: Wiley-Blackwell.
Housley, W. (2000). Category work and knowledgeability within multidisciplinary team meetings. *Text, 20*(1), 83–107.
Houtkoop, H. (1987). *Establishing agreement: An analysis of proposal-acceptance sequences*. Dordrecht, NL: Foris Publications.
Huisman, M. (2001). Decision-making in meetings as talk-in-interaction. *International Studies of Management & Organization, 31*(3), 69–90.
Ijäs-Kallio, T., Ruusuvuori, J., & Peräkylä, A. (2011). 'Unilateral' decision making and patient participation in primary care. *Communication & Medicine, 8*(2), 145–155.
Kangasharju, H. (1996). Aligning as a team in multiparty conversation. *Journal of Pragmatics, 26*(3), 291–319.
Kangasharju, H. (2002). Alignment in disagreement: Forming oppositional alliances in committee meetings. *Journal of Pragmatics, 34*(10), 1447–1471.

Knapp, M. (2003). Hidden costs of mental illness. *The British Journal of Psychiatry, 183*(6), 477–478.

Koenig, C. J. (2011). Patient resistance as agency in treatment decisions. *Social Science and Medicine, 72*(7), 1105–1114.

Krummheuer, A. (2020). Instrumental and moral assistance: An embodied interaction analysis of assisted shopping activities between a person with acquired brain injury and her caregivers. *Pragmatics and Society, 11*(3), 439–461.

Kushida, S., & Yamakawa, Y. (2015). Fitting proposals to their sequential environment: A comparison of turn designs for proposing treatment in ongoing outpatient psychiatric consultations in Japan. *Sociology of Health & Illness, 37*(4), 522–544.

Laakso, M. (1997). *Self-initiated repair by fluent aphasic speakers in conversation*. Helsinki: Finnish Literature Society.

Larquet, M., Coricelli, G., Opolczynski, G., & Thibaut, F. (2010). Impaired decision making in schizophrenia and orbitofrontal cortex lesion patients. *Schizophrenia Research, 116*(2), 266–273.

LeBlanc, H. P. (2018). Communicating inclusion: An analysis of family conversation. *International Journal of Linguistics & Communication, 6*(2), 1–11.

Lerner, G. (1996). On the place of linguistic resources in the organization of talk-in-interaction: 'Second-person' reference in multi-party conversation. *Pragmatics, 6,* 281–294.

Levinson, S. C. (2013). Action formation and ascription. In J. Sidnell & T. Stivers (Eds.), *Handbook of conversation analysis* (pp. 103–130). Boston, MA: Wiley-Blackwell.

Liddicoat, A. J. (2011). *An introduction to conversation analysis.* London: Continuum.

Lindholm, C. (2015). Parallel realities: The interactional management of confabulation in dementia care encounters. *Research on Language and Social Interaction, 48*(2), 176–199.

Lindholm, C., & Stevanovic, M. (2020/in press). Challenges of trust in atypical interaction. *Pragmatics and Society.*

Lindström, A., & Weatherall, A. (2015). Orientations to epistemics and deontics in treatment discussions. *Journal of Pragmatics, 78,* 39–53.

Linell, P. (1998). *Approaching dialogue: Talk, interaction and contexts in dialogical perspectives*. Amsterdam: Benjamins.

Linell, P., & Luckmann, T. (1991). Asymmetries in dialogue: Some conceptual preliminaries. In I. Markova & K. Foppa (Eds.), *Asymmetries in dialogue* (pp. 1–20). Hemel Hempstead: Harvester.

Loh, A., Simon, D., Wills, C. E., Kriston, L., Niebling, W., & Härter, M. (2007). The effects of a shared decision-making intervention in primary

care of depression: A cluster-randomized controlled trial. *Patient Education and Counseling, 67*(3), 324–332.
Marshall, T. H. (1964). *Class, citizenship, and social development.* Chicago: University of Chicago Press.
Maynard, D. W. (1984). *Inside plea bargaining: The language of negotiation.* New York: Plenum.
Maynard, D. W. (2005). Social actions, gestalt coherence, and designations of disability: Lessons from and about autism. *Social Problems, 52*(4), 499–524.
McCabe, R., & Healey, P. (2018). Miscommunication in doctor-patient communication. *Topics in Cognitive Science, 10*(2), 409–424.
McCabe, R., Heath, C., Burns, T., & Priebe, S. (2002). Engagement of patients with psychosis in the consultation. *British Medical Journal, 325,* 1148–1151.
McCabe, R., & Lavelle, M. (2012). Participation in multiparty interaction: A single case analysis of a patient with schizophrenia. *Proceedings of Video Analysis on Work, Interaction and Technology: A Festschrift for Christian Heath. Bayreuth, Landratesaal,* 97–108.
Mikesell, L. (2009). Conversational practices of a frontotemporal dementia patient and his interlocutors. *Research on Language and Social Interaction, 42*(2), 135–162.
Morgan, C., Burns, T., Fitzpatrick, R., Pinfold, V., & Priebe, S. (2007). Social exclusion and mental health: Conceptual and methodological review. *The British Journal of Psychiatry, 191*(6), 477–483.
Mundwiler, V., & Kreuz, J. (2018). Collaborative decision-making in argumentative group discussions among primary school children. In S. Oswald, T. Herman, & J. Jacquin (Eds.), *Argumentation and language—Linguistic, cognitive and discursive explorations* (pp. 263–285). Cham: Springer.
Nissi, R. (2015). From entry proposals to a joint statement: Practices of shared text production in multiparty meeting interaction. *Journal of Pragmatics, 79,* 1–21.
O'Donovan, A. (2007). Patient-centred care in acute psychiatric admission units: Reality or rhetoric? *Journal of Psychiatric and Mental Health Nursing, 14*(6), 542–548.
Osborne, S. P., & Strokosch, K. (2013). It takes two to tango? Understanding the co-production of public services by integrating the services management and public administration perspectives. *British Journal of Management, 24*(S1), S31–S47.
Pateman, C. (1970). *Participation and democratic theory.* Cambridge: Cambridge University Press.

Payne, S. (2006). Mental health, poverty and social exclusion. In C. Pantazis, D. Gordon, & R. Levitas (Eds.), *Poverty and social exclusion in Britain: The millennium survey* (pp. 285–311). Bristol: Policy Press.

Peräkylä, A. (1995). *AIDS counselling: Institutional interaction and clinical practice*. Cambridge: Cambridge University Press.

Pilnick, A., & Coleman, T. (2003). 'I'll give up smoking when you get me better': Patients' resistance to attempts to problematise smoking in general practice (GP) consultations. *Social Science and Medicine, 57*(1), 135–145.

Pomerantz, A. (1984). Agreeing and disagreeing with assessments: Some features of preferred/dispreferred turn shaped. In J. M. Atkinson & J. Heritage (Eds.), *Structures of social action* (pp. 57–101). Cambridge: Cambridge University Press.

Quirk, A., Chapin, R., Lelliott, P., & Seale, C. (2012). How pressure is applied in shared decisions about antipsychotic medication: A conversation analytic study of psychiatric outpatient consultations. *Sociology of Health & Illness, 34*(1), 95–113.

Raymond, G., & Heritage, J. (2006). The epistemics of social relations: Owning grandchildren. *Language in Society, 35*(5), 677–705.

Rissmiller, D. J., & Rissmiller, J. H. (2006). Open forum: Evolution of the antipsychiatry movement into mental health consumerism. *Psychiatric Services, 57*(6), 863–866.

Robinson, J. D. (2001). Asymmetry in action: Sequential resources in the negotiation of a prescription request. *Text, 21*(1–2), 19–54.

Roter, D. (2000). The enduring and evolving nature of the patient–physician relationship. *Patient Education and Counseling, 39*(1), 5–15.

Royal College of Psychiatrists Social Inclusion Scoping Group. (2009). *Mental health and social inclusion: Making psychiatry and mental health services fit for the 21st century*. Position Statement PS01/2009. https://www.rcpsych.ac.uk/docs/default-source/mental-health/work-and-mental-health-library/position-statement-2009.pdf?sfvrsn=97bca29e_2.

Ruusuvuori, J. (2000). *Control in medical consultation: Practices for giving and receiving the reason for the visit in primary health care*. Tampere: University of Tampere.

Sacks, H., Schegloff, E. A., & Jefferson, G. (1974). A simplest systematics for the organization of turn-taking for conversation. *Language, 50*(4), 696–735.

Schegloff, E. A. (1995). Discourse as an interactional achievement III: The omnirelevance of action. *Research on Language and Social Interaction, 28*(3), 185–211.

Schegloff, E. A. (1996). Some practices of referring to persons in talk-in-interaction: A partial sketch of a systematics. In B. Fox (Ed.), *Studies in anaphora* (pp. 437–485). Amsterdam: Benjamins.
Schegloff, E. A. (2007). *Sequence organization in interaction.* Cambridge: Cambridge University Press.
Schegloff, E. A., Jefferson, G., & Sacks, H. (1977). The preference for self-correction in the organization of repair in conversation. *Language, 53,* 361–382.
Schegloff, E. A., & Sacks, H. (1973). Opening up closings. *Semiotica, 8*(4), 289–327.
Sihvo, S., Isola, A.-M., Kivipelto, M. Linnanmäki, E., Lyytikäinen, M., & Sainio, S. (2018). *Operating model for client involvement.* Reports and Memorandums of the Ministry of Social Affairs and Health 16/2018. http://julkaisut.valtioneuvosto.fi/handle/10024/160828.
Slade, M. (2017). Implementing shared decision making in routine mental health care. *World Psychiatry, 16*(2), 146–153.
Stevanovic, M. (2012). Establishing joint decisions in a dyad. *Discourse Studies, 14*(6), 779–803.
Stevanovic, M. (2013). Deontic rights in interaction: A conversation analytic study on authority and cooperation. *Publications of the Department of Social Research* 2013:10. University of Helsinki. https://helda.helsinki.fi/bitstream/handle/10138/39270/stevanovic_dissertation.pdf?sequence=1.
Stevanovic, M. (2018). Social deontics: A nano-level approach to human power play. *Journal for the Theory of Social Behaviour, 48*(3), 369–389.
Stevanovic, M., Henttonen, P., Koski, S., Kahri, M., Voutilainen, L., Koskinen, E., ... Peräkylä, A. (2017). On the Asperger experience of interaction: Interpersonal dynamics in dyadic conversations. *Journal of Autism, 4*(2), http://www.hoajonline.com/autism/2054-992X/4/2.
Stevanovic, M., Lehtinen, E., Lindholm, C., Nissi, R., Valkeapää, T., & Weiste, E. (forthcoming). Vuorovaikutus, osallistuminen ja tekstin yhteinen tuottaminen: Tapaustutkimus valmennusryhmäkeskusteluista [Interaction, participation and the joint construction of text: A case study of group counselling conversations].
Stevanovic, M., & Peräkylä, A. (2012). Deontic authority in interaction: The right to announce, propose and decide. *Research on Language and Social Interaction, 45*(3), 297–321.
Stevanovic, M., & Svennevig, J. (2015). Introduction: Epistemics and deontics in conversational directives. *Journal of Pragmatics, 78,* 1–6.

Stevanovic, M., Valkeapää, T., Weiste, E., & Lindholm, C. (2020/in press). Joint decision making in a mental health rehabilitation community: The impact of support workers' proposal design on client responsiveness. *Counselling Psychology Quarterly*.
Stivers, T. (2005). Parent resistance to physicians' treatment recommendations: One resource for initiating a negotiation of the treatment decision. *Health Communication, 18*(1), 41–74.
Stivers, T. (2006). Treatment decisions: Negotiations between doctors and parents in acute care encounters. In J. Heritage & D. W. Maynard (Eds.), *Communication in medical care: Interaction between primary care physicians and patients* (pp. 279–312). Cambridge: Cambridge University Press.
Stivers, T., Heritage, J., Barnes, R. K., McCabe, R., Thompson, L., & Toerien, M. (2018). Treatment recommendations as actions. *Health Communication, 33*(11), 1335–1344.
Stivers, T., & Rossano, F. (2010). Mobilizing response. *Research on Language and Social Interaction, 43*(1), 3–31.
Stovell, D., Morrison, A. P., Panayiotou, M., & Hutton, P. (2016). Shared treatment decision-making and empowerment-related outcomes in psychosis: Systematic review and meta-analysis. *The British Journal of Psychiatry, 209*(1), 23–28.
Tambuyzer, E., Pieters, G., & Van Audenhove, C. (2014). Patient involvement in mental health care: one size does not fit all. *Health Expectations, 17*(1), 138–150.
Tannen, D. (2005). *Conversational style: Analyzing talk among friends*. New York: Oxford University Press.
ten Have, P. (2007). *Doing conversation analysis: A practical guide*. London: Sage.
Thompson, A. G. (2007). The meaning of patient involvement and participation in health care consultations: A taxonomy. *Social Science and Medicine, 64*(6), 1297–1310.
Thompson, L., & McCabe, R. (2018). How psychiatrists recommend treatment and its relationship with patient uptake. *Health Communication, 33*(11), 1345–1354.
Toerien, M., Shaw, R., & Reuber, M. (2013). Initiating decision-making in neurology consultations: 'Recommending' versus 'option-listing' and the implications for medical authority. *Sociology of Health & Illness, 35*(6), 873–890.

Treichler, E. B., & Spaulding, W. D. (2017). Beyond shared decision-making: Collaboration in the age of recovery from serious mental illness. *American Journal of Orthopsychiatry, 87*(5), 567–574.

Volk, R. J., Shokar, N. K., Leal, V. B., Bulik, R. J., Linder, S. K., Mullen, P. D., ... Shokar, G. S. (2014). Development and pilot testing of an online case-based approach to shared decision making skills training for clinicians. *BMC Medical Informatics and Decision Making, 14*(1), 95.

Walker, E. (1995). Making a bid for change: Formulations in union/management negotiations. In A. Firth (Ed.), *The discourse of negotiation: Studies of language in the workplace* (pp. 101–140). Oxford: Pergamon.

Weiste, E., Peräkylä, A., Valkeapää, T., Savander, E., & Hintikka, J. (2018). Institutionalised otherness: Patients references to psychiatric diagnostic categories. *Social Science & Medicine, 207*, 71–79.

Weiste, E., Voutilainen, L., & Peräkylä, A. (2016). Epistemic asymmetries in psychotherapy interaction: Therapists' practices for displaying access to clients' inner experiences. *Sociology of Health & Illness, 38*(4), 645–661.

Whalen, J., Zimmerman, D. H., & Whalen, M. R. (1988). When words fail: A single case analysis. *Social Problems, 35*(4), 335–362.

WHO. (2013). *Mental health action plan 2013–2020.* Geneva: WHO Press. http://apps.who.int/iris/bitstream/handle/10665/89966/9789241506021_eng.pdf;jsessionid=0767FE6F65666AD0F15661CD9613EDFC?sequence=1.

2

Promoting Client Participation and Constructing Decisions in Mental Health Rehabilitation Meetings

Melisa Stevanovic, Taina Valkeapää, Elina Weiste, and Camilla Lindholm

One key form of participation is the right to make joint decisions. In recent decades, the importance of joint decision-making has been highlighted in the field of social and health care, where the client's right to self-determination and empowerment have been emphasized (Epstein et al., 2005). In mental health care, particularly in the United States since the 1970s, this development has been influenced by the political movement of mental health client groups seeking to improve their position and raising the

M. Stevanovic (✉) · T. Valkeapää
University of Helsinki, Helsinki, Finland
e-mail: melisa.stevanovic@helsinki.fi

T. Valkeapää
e-mail: taina.valkeapaa@helsinki.fi

E. Weiste
Finnish Institute of Occupational Health, Helsinki, Finland
e-mail: elina.weiste@ttl.fi

C. Lindholm
Tampere University, Tampere, Finland
e-mail: camilla.lindholm@tuni.fi

C. Lindholm et al. (eds.), *Joint Decision Making in Mental Health*,
The Language of Mental Health, https://doi.org/10.1007/978-3-030-43531-8_2

right to decision-making as a matter of human rights (Chamberlin, 1990; Drake, Deegan, & Rapp, 2010). The ideals of "shared decision-making" (Barry & Edgman-Levitan, 2012; Charles, Gafni, & Whelan, 1999) and "collaborative decision-making" (Treichler & Spaulding, 2017) have later become key concepts informing the client care practices.

In mental health care, the realization of the shared and collaborative decision-making ideals has turned out to be particularly challenging. Some of these challenges have been related to deficits in the individual decision-making capacities of mental health clients (see Beitinger, Kissling, & Hamann, 2014; Ernst & Paulus, 2005; Larquet, Coricelli, Opolczynski, & Thibaut, 2010). Furthermore, some clients have explicitly expressed a wish to leave the decisions about their own treatment in the hands of professionals only (Elstad & Eide, 2009; Hickey & Kipping, 1998). As a result, many professionals' attempts to promote client participation are met with some degree of client passivity or resistance. In this chapter, we analyze decision-making sequences in a setting where these kinds of challenges are apparent, while we focus on the support workers' practices of dealing with these challenges.

Constructing the Outcome of Decision-Making as a "Joint" Decision

Joint decision-making is not only a matter of participants distributing their activities during the decision-making process so that each of them has a "share" in it, based on each participant's specific domain of knowledge or expertise. In addition, the construction of the outcome of decision-making as a "joint" decision necessitates that the participants also constantly negotiate the status of their shared activity as a joint decision-making activity. These negotiations not only concern the *content* of the decisions to be made, but also *whether*, *when*, and *on what exactly* the participants are making decisions about in the first place.

Stevanovic (2012) has elucidated these multiple levels of joint decision-making with reference to three components of an accepting or approving response to a proposal. When formulating their ideas about future actions or events as proposals, and not as order or announcements, the speaker treats their co-participants as having a word to say in the realization of these ideas. A proposal can therefore be considered to be the starting point of a joint decision-making sequence. It is then the ways in which the other participants present respond to the proposal that lead the sequence either toward a decision or toward something else. According to Stevanovic (2012), in order to establish a joint decision, the recipients of a proposal need to claim understanding of what the proposal is about (*access*), indicate that the proposed plan is feasible (*agreement*), and demonstrate willingness to treat the plan as binding (*commitment*). Essentially, it is the recipients of the proposal who bear the main responsibility for taking the decision-making sequence forward. This orientation allows the proposal recipient to avoid explicit rejection of proposals, since instead, they can abandon the sequence before a decision has been established (see also Stevanovic, 2015). If the proposer instead pushes the sequence forward, for example, by actively pursuing a response from the recipients, the genuine jointness of the decision-making outcome is compromised. In this way, the nature of any decision-making outcome is a result of the moment-by-moment sequential unfolding of the decision-making process (Fig. 2.1).

The right to propose and decide is a central manifestation of the so-called "deontic authority" (Stevanovic & Peräkylä, 2012). From this perspective, the trajectories of sequences from proposals to the displays of access, agreement, and commitment are also a matter of maintaining equality in terms of a symmetrical distribution of power. As Stevanovic (2012, 2015) has argued, establishing such a symmetry can be facilitated by all participants orienting to the responsibility

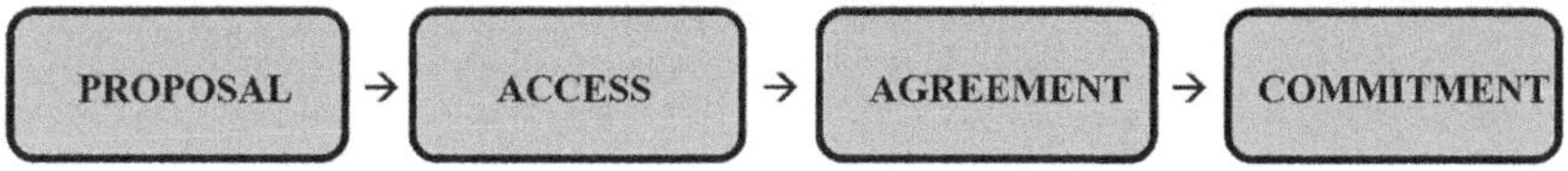

Fig. 2.1 Components of the joint decision-making sequence (Stevanovic, 2012)

of the recipients in determining the ultimate destiny of the given proposal. But what happens when the recipients may not be trusted to take on this responsibility? This question is what this chapter seeks to illuminate.

The Research Context

This study was conducted in the context of mental health rehabilitation at the Clubhouse. The Clubhouse movement started in New York in the 1940s, when mental health patients sought to reduce the isolation associated with mental health problems by organizing various communal activities (Hänninen, 2016). Today, the activities at Clubhouse communities are based on the international Clubhouse model, which seeks to improve mental health clients' quality of life, reduce their need of hospital care, and support their return to work (Hänninen, 2016). In Finland, the Clubhouse is a third-sector player in the mental health rehabilitation service system. Clubhouse communities can be joined without a referral by a mental health professional, but workers at psychiatric hospitals or outpatient clinics typically encourage clients to contact these communities when the rehabilitation process is to be prolonged and the client's ability to work and functional capacities are threatened.

Clubhouse communities involve both mental health clients and support workers. Clients are called members, and membership of a Clubhouse community is understood to mean that members have the right and obligation to participate in decision-making about communal life. Such an understanding is also in line with the so-called "recovery approach" (Davidson, O'Connell, Tondora, Lawless, & Evans, 2005; Hänninen, 2012), which has criticized the traditional medical model of mental illness for its excessive professionalism and promoted an equal relationship between professionals and clients.

Research Question

Given the status of joint decision-making as an explicit ideal of the Clubhouse model on one hand, and the passivity or resistance that often characterizes the behavior of mental health clients in joint decision-making contexts on the other, in this paper we seek to illuminate the interactional details of this discrepancy. We ask: what are the practices through which support workers at the Clubhouse seek to encourage the clients to contribute to joint decision-making sequences?

Data and Method

The data for this study were collected at one Finnish Clubhouse in 2016–2017. Our material consists of weekly video-recorded group meetings of mental health clients and support workers, at which the clients sought to practice their working life skills. The dataset contains a total of 29 meetings, while their duration varied between 30 and 70 min. Each meeting involved 2–10 clients and 1–3 support workers, who had undertaken professional training in social work. During the meetings, a wide range of decisions was made, most of which concerned the activities of the group. The names and other participant identifiers used in the analysis of the data transcripts have been anonymized. Transcription symbols and glossing abbreviations are provided in the Appendix. Our method of investigation was conversation analysis (Sacks & Schegloff, 1973; Schegloff, 2007; Sidnell, 2013), which seeks to unravel the resources through which everyday social life is built (for a more extended discussion, see Chapter 1).

Analysis: Practices to Promote Participation and Construct Decisions

In this section, we account for the variation of the support workers' practices across our data collection. In so doing, we use the above-described model of joint decision-making (Stevanovic, 2012).

Retrospective Construction of Proposals

As pointed out, the starting point of joint decision-making involves one participant making a proposal for a future action or event. From the perspective of deontic authority, the mere act of making a proposal involves a claim of the right to have a word to say in what will be done. From this it follows that a substantial level of client participation could be immediately achieved if it were the *clients*, and not the support workers, who produced the proposals. In the face of a relative scarcity of client proposals in our data (cf. Chapter 6), support workers occasionally seem to engage in remarkable interactional work to emphasize those elements in the clients' prior talk that could be interpreted as suggestive of plans.

Extract 1a is from a situation where the participants are planning the program for the entire autumn season. Previously, one of the support workers (SW1) has listed the themes discussed by that group during the spring. As one such theme, she has mentioned an activity that involved the group members making plans for their own rehabilitation. At the beginning of Extract 1a she shifts the discussion to the current situation, when the group should decide what to do next (line 1).

Extract 1a

01 SW1: ↑mutta (.) mitä me tehään ↑tästä eteenpäin.
but (.) what shall we do from now on.

02 (7.0)

03 Aki: **nii onks sitä ny (.) varsinaisesti, (0.2)**
P be-Q it-PAR P actually
yeah has it been now (.) actually, (0.2)

04 **otettu, (1.0) ninku, (0.5) realisoitu sitä**
take-PPPC P realize-PPPC it-PAR
taken up, (1.0) like, (0.5) realized it

05 **et et et (.) hh näitä ↑toteutettu mi-**
CP CP PC these-PAR realize-PPPC
so that (.) these (would have been) realized

06 **mist on puhuttu (0.4) vai.**
what-PAR be talk-PPPC or
that we have been talking about (0.4) or.

07 (1.0)

08 SW1: nii et (.) tarkotaksä et niit tavotteita jotka
yeah so (.) do you mean those goals that

09 jokainen asetti sit siellä,
everyone set there,

10 Aki: ↑nii nii ja siis noita että ku tos on noita
yea yea and I mean those that since there are those

11 omien rajojen tunnistaminen
recognizing one's limits

12 stressinsietoo ja tommosii nii jos niitä,
stress resilience and the like so I wonder if these

13 (0.3) niitä ↑testattu tai (.) kokeiltu tai
(0.3) have been tested or (.) tried or

```
14        ninku että just Anu sano et te olitte tehny
          like Anu just said that you had done

15        kokeillu uusii et onko, (1.0) onko sitte,
          tried some new so has, (1.0) has there then been,

16        (0.5) (-) (1.0) ketkä täs nyt on jo sitte
          (0.5) (-) (1.0) who have now already

17        ↑kokeillu kaikkia erilaisia (.) (--)
          tried all kinds of different (.) (--)

18        kiinnostavia hommia,
          interesting stuff,

19        (1.0)

20 SW1:   no se on jäänytietenki vähänninku
          well it has of course been left sort of like

21        jokaisen omalle vastuulle
          to everyone's own responsibility
```

After SW1's open question (line 1), a long silence ensues (line 2). Finally, one of the clients, Aki, takes a turn, asking if the plans made last spring have been implemented (lines 3–6). We interpret Aki's turn as an indirect critical statement about the group's activities in general—about there being "a lot of talk, but little action." The breaks and restarts in Aki's turn, which indicate interactional difficulties, support the interpretation. After a silence (line 7), SW1 requests Aki to clarify his turn (lines 8–9), which he then does in lines 10–18. Similar to Aki's original turn, his subsequent clarification turn also entails elements that appear critical of the group's activities ("I wonder if these have been tested," lines 12–13). This is also how SW1 orients to Aki's turn as action: after a silence in line 19, she starts to defend the group's activities (lines 20–21). By appealing to each group member's "own responsibility" for the implementation of their plans, SW1 evades the implied criticism that this would have needed to be done by the group.

A moment later, however, Aki's action will be dealt with in another way. In the meanwhile, just before Extract 1b, the group has decided that one of the clients, Noa, will act as the meeting secretary (lines 40–49, not shown in the transcript). Noa, therefore, needs to know what to write in the meeting minutes. Thus, as part of a clarification for Noa in this respect, the other support worker (SW2), who was silent during Extract 1a, makes a reference to Aki's previous talk (lines 50–51).

Extract 1b

50 SW2: ku mä aattelin et **tässähän tuli nyt**
P SG1 think-1 CP here-CLI come-PST now
because I was thinking that **here there just came**

51 **yksi**, (.) **yks idea Akilla** (.) (--)
one one idea MaleName-ADE
one, (.) **one idea by Aki** (.) (--)

52 laittaa vähän ranskiksilla sinne ylös (-)
(we should) write down some bullet points (-)

53 voidaan sit miettiä,
we can then think about (them),

54 Noa: mikäs se [oli.
what was [it

55 SW2: [elikkä, (1.2) sulla oli vähän ninku
[so, (1.2) you had sort of like

56 sitä (.) <oman toiminnan arviointia>
that (.) evaluation of one's own action

57 (.)

```
58 Aki: nii [tai nii nii siis mitä tuolta kattoo muuta    ]
        yea [or yea yea I mean what else you can see there]

59 SW2:     [näitten pohjalta työnkuvan arviointi         ]
            [evaluation of profile on the basis of these]

60 Aki: että jos ninku, (0.8) sillee että (.)
        so that if (it is) like, (0.8) so that (.)

61      ninku nyt Maisaki just sano et tekemällä oppii
        like Maisa now just said that you learn by doing

62      ni (.) siin sitte, (0.8) et, (0.5)
        so (.) there then, (0.8) that, (0.5)

63      ite en oo niin (.) noist
        I myself am not that (much) into (.) the kind of

64      (.) teoriajutuista niin,
        (.) theory stuff so,
```

Instead of orienting to Aki's previous talk as a critical statement, SW2 treats it as a proposal: Aki has suggested an "idea" (lines 50–51) that Noa should write down (lines 52–53). Next, Noa asks what Aki's idea was (line 54), which is then responded to by SW2 formulating Aki's idea as a call for the group to engage in some sort of evaluation activities (lines 55–56, 59). Thereafter, Aki takes a turn. The repetitive elements in his turn-beginning ("yea or yea yea I mean," line 58) imply a need for an adjustment to the support worker's prior turn. Instead of explicitly rejecting SW2's interpretation of his previous action, Aki makes a reference to Maisa, who has previously emphasized the importance of practical action instead of "theory stuff" (line 60–64). Thus, while Aki basically repeats his previous point about what may not be optimal in the activities of the group, the element of criticism becomes transformed into an expression of personal preference—something that may also inform the decisions to be made. In this way, Aki has ultimately become an active participant in joint decision-making.

Reminding About Access

Evidently, a mere proposal is not enough to establish a joint decision. Instead, as pointed out above, a joint decision requires that the recipients of the proposal work to move the sequence forwards toward the decision. The first component of such approving responses to proposals involves a display of *access* to the content of the proposal. When the recipients fail to recognize what the proposal is about, sometimes it may lead to a de facto rejection of the proposal, without this rejection ever surfacing at the level of participants' explicit talk. This interactionally easy and face-saving way of rejecting a proposal is nonetheless dependent on the proposer refraining from pursuing the same proposal anymore.

However, what we observed in our data was that in the face of a lack of recipient uptake, the support workers did *not* abandon their proposals but, instead sought to remind the recipients of their access to the content of the proposal. Extract 2a is a case in point. Previously, one of the support workers (SW2) has mentioned a theme that the group has dealt with at its previous meetings during spring. Now, she suggests that the same theme could also be discussed during the autumn. However, she presents her idea as contingent on the group not experiencing it as excessive repetition (lines 1–7, 9).

Extract 2a

```
01 SW2: mä aattelin et nyt täs on seuraava (.) aihe
        I thought that now here we have the next (.) theme

((lines 2-5 removed))

06      ne on nyt varmaan aika pitkälti siis samantyyppisiä
        now they are certainly to a large extent similar

07      ku tä[ä  e]t mä mietin (.) nyt sitäkin että
        to th[is s]o I wonder (.) now also if

08 SW1:      [mm,]
             [mm,]
```

```
09 SW2: tuleeks siit ke:rtausta sitte,
        there will be too much repetition then,

10      (0.7)

11 SW1: mut se ↑näkökulma ↑voi olla >vähä< erilaine↑,
        but the perspective can be somewhat different

12      (0.4) miltä se tu- kuulostaa.
        (0.4) how does it sound.

13 SW2: ni,=
        so,=

14 SW1: =haittaako vaikka tulee kertausta,
        =do you mind if there will be repetition,

15      (3.0)

16 SW1: ne   jotka on keväällä   ollu   näit
        they who  be spring-ADE be-PPC these-PAR
        those who were thinking about these

17      pohtimassa    mitä sanotte.
        think-INF-INE what say-PL2
        in the Spring what do you say.

18      (0.4)

19 SW1: Make     tai Sini       tai Ai[ri.]
        MaleName or FemaleName or FemaleName
        Make     or Sini       or Ai[ri.]
```

After SW2's question (line 9), there is a short silence (line 10), after which her co-worker (SW1) supports the idea by pointing out the possible different perspectives to the same theme (lines 11). Thereafter, SW1 requests the group members to take a stance toward the idea: first she poses an open question (line 12) and then a polar question, asking the group members whether they regard repetition as a problem (line 14). Given that both support workers at the meeting have already taken a stance toward the idea, it is obvious that it is the clients who have been addressed by the question. However, none of them reacts. Thus, after a three-second silence (line 15), SW1 directs the question to those clients who, could be expected to know exactly what the proposal is about, based on their earlier membership in the group (lines 16–17, 19). In so doing, SW1 reminds the clients about their epistemic access to the content of the proposal. As can be seen in Extract 2b, this support worker's attempt is successful in encouraging client response (see lines 20–22, 24–25 & 28).

Extract 2b

20 Ada: **[ei] hai[ttaa].**
[I] don't [mind].

21 Mio: **[ei h]aittaa.**
[I do]n't mind.

22 **m- mäki kävin sillon kevää[llä] jo.**
I also was there in the Sp[ring] already.

23 SW1: [ni.]
[yea.]

24 Ada: **ei haittaa.**
I don't mind.

25 Kim: joo,
yea,

26 (1.0)

27 SW1: ↑no ni,
↑okay,

28 (3.0) **((Sini nods.))**

29 Kim: .mt **mä oon vissiin yks (.) yks jääny väliin.**
SG1 be-1 surely one one leave-PPC between
.mt I guess I have missed one (.) one

30 (1.2)

31 Kim: **(vain.)**
(only.)

32 SW2: °okei,°
°okay,°

33 Ada: .thh **mullakaan ei oo pahemmin**
SG1-ADE-CLI NEG be bad-ADV-COMP
.thh **neither do I have many**

Despite the matter that several clients now give a preferred answer to the support worker's polar question about whether the realization of the proposal would be a problem, the further unfolding of the sequence deviates from the trajectory of joint decision-making. Instead of working to establish a joint decision, the clients topicalize the source of their epistemic access to the content of the proposal—they discuss how often each of them has been absent from the group meetings during spring (lines 29, 31 & 33). Thus, although an orientation to and a public display of access to the content of a proposal takes the decision-making sequence substantially forward from the mere stating of a proposal, from the perspective of keeping the focus of discussion on joint decision-making, the act of reminding others about their epistemic access is a risky endeavor. This is because it topicalizes something that is only tangential to the actual proposal content.

More importantly, however, the support workers' insisting on active client participation, paradoxically, compromised the genuine jointness of the decision-making outcome. In giving the clients no option *not* to respond to the proposal, the clients could not use silence as a way to convey reluctance or a lack of interest toward what was being proposed. In this way, the clients lost the options (1) to indicate a rejection of the proposal in an easy and face-saving way and (2) to influence the meta-level decision on whether the idea should be decided on in the first place.

Pursuing Agreement

In addition to reminding participants about their epistemic access to the content of the proposal, proposers may sometimes pursue their co-participants' agreement with their ideas quite straightforwardly. This is what happens in Extract 3a, where the participants discuss the so-called "transitional work"—a Clubhouse-created employment program, the aim of which is to assist those Clubhouse members who wish to seek competitive employment in the future. It involves a part-time placement at the employer's place of business, lasting from 6 to 9 months (Valkeapää, Lindholm, Tanaka, Weiste, & Stevanovic, 2019).

Here, a support worker (SW1) suggests that a group of Clubhouse members from another community could visit the group to report their experiences of transitional work (lines 1–7; lines 3–7 not shown in the transcript).

Extract 3a

01 SW1: no ↑mitäs te sanotte sit semmoseen
well what do you say to the kind of (idea) that

02 ku meillähän ↑kävi sitte tossa,
you know we had (those visitors)

((lines 3-7 removed))

08 Kai: mä oli siinä (-)=
I was there (-)=

09 SW1: =↑no ↑sä olit ↑ainaki. (.)
=↑so ↑at least ↑you were there. (.)

10 mimmonen se sun mielest oli se juttu,
how was it in your opinion,

11 Kai: no kylhän se (--) kumminki (.) saa vähä
well surely it (--) anyway (.) one gets some

12 tietoo tota noin noist (.) ee paikoista ja,
information erm about those (.) ee places and,

13 SW1: mm,
mm,

14 Kai: tämmöstä mitä siihen vaaditaan ja tämmös[tä::,]
kind of what is demanded for that and th[e kind]

15 SW1: [mm-m,]

16 (.)

17 Kai: semmosta.
sort of.

18 SW1: **jaksaisiksä kuunnella sellast**
be.able.to-COND-2+SG2 listen-INF that.kind.of-PAR
could you bear listening to that kind of (talk)

```
19          toisteki.
            another.time-CLI
            also another time.

20 Kai:     no::, (0.5) kyl ↑mä ↑varmaan jaksaisin.
            P           P   SG1 I.guess  be.able.to-COND-2
            we::ll, (0.5) yes I guess I could bear that.

21          ((general laughter))

22 SW1:     kiva.
            nice.
```

In response to SW1's proposal (lines 1–7), Kai reminds others about him having been present at a previous similar event, thus displaying access to the content of the proposal (line 8). Kai, however, refrains from providing any assessment of his experience. Thus, after acknowledging Kai's past presence in the event (line 9), SW1 asks for Kai's assessment of it ("how was it in your opinion," line 10). Kai responds, again refraining from taking a clear position in favor of or against the proposed idea. The positive start of the turn (*no kylhän se* "well surely it," line 11) implies that the usefulness of the event is not to be taken for granted (Niemi, 2010). In the continuation of the turn, Kai states that the event was able to provide him "some information" but he refrains from any evaluation of the usefulness of that information (lines 11–12, 14, 17).

While Kai's lack of evaluation of the event could be considered meaningful, this is not the way SW1 treats Kai's turn. Shifting the focus from the past event to a possible analogous future event, she poses a polar question to Kai, which requires him to take a clear position on the proposal ("could you bear listening to that kind of (talk) also another time," lines 18–19). In response to this, Kai produces a somewhat evasive answer ("we::ll, (0.5) yes I guess I could bear that," line 20), where the long-stretched Finnish particle *no* "well" implies some difficulty in producing the answer and the repetition of the verb "bear," which SW1 has (possibly ironically) used in her question, implies that what SW1 has proposed is indeed something that requires "bearing" from him. The other members of the group laugh at Kai's answer (line 21), thus treating it primarily as humor. SW1, nonetheless, seems to treat Kai's response as an acceptance of her proposal: in response to Kai's turn, she utters an evaluative token *kiva* "nice" (line 22), after which a new topic is launched.

Later during the same meeting, the other support worker present at the meeting (SW2) briefly refers to the idea of visitors (lines 73–75, 77 & 79).

Extract 3b

71 SW2: ↑voidaanhan me käydä esimerkiks joku kerta
certainly we could have sometime

72 sellanen (.) keskustelu että että tota (.)
the kind of (.) discussion that that erm (.)

73 **vaikka sillon jos tulee näitäkin (.) jäseniä**
P then if come these-CLI member-PL-PAR
for example then if there will be those (.) members

74 **jotka on, (0.3) sieltä kaupungista**
who-PL be from.there city-ELA
who are, (0.3) from that city

75 **[jotka] on, (0.3) on tota noin niin**
who-PL be be P P P
[who] have, (0.3) have erm

76 SW1: [mm-m,]
[mm-m,]

77 SW2: **käyny [sen,]**
completed [that,]

78 SW1: [mm-m] mm-m,
[mm-m] mm-m,

79 SW2: **tehny siirtymätyöjaksoja** (.)
done transitional work periods (.)

80 ja sitten meillä on
and then we have

In Extract 3b, SW2 refers to the possibility of having visitors, but she does not invite new discussions on the matter. Instead, the reference to the visitors is embedded in a discussion about the group's schedule (lines 71–73). The ultimate decision on whether to invite visitors is thus treated as open (see the particle *jos* "if," line 73), while the very group in the here and now is *not* treated as the *maker* of that ultimate decision.

As suggested at the beginning of the chapter, the matter that the proposal recipients "voluntarily" take a stance in favor of a proposal serves as a warrant for the substantiality of their acceptance of the proposal, which is a precondition for constructing the outcome of the sequence as a *joint* decision. Voluntariness, however, necessitates that the recipients also have an actual option to refrain from taking such a stance and, in so doing, prevent the sequence from proceeding toward a decision. Thus, the proposer's act of encouraging stance-taking from the proposal recipients has the paradoxical consequence of leading the sequence to an interactional outcome other than a genuinely joint decision.

Pursuing Commitment and Establishing Decisions

As suggested before, a joint decision is established when the recipients of the proposal have expressed their commitment to the proposed action. If the recipients refrain from doing so, the proposer may either abandon the sequence, thus acknowledging the lack of commitment as meaningful, or seek to encourage the recipients' commitment, thus risking the jointness of the decision-making outcome. The latter option is pursued in the example below, in which the group has previously discussed how the group should be named. At the beginning of the extract, one of the support workers (SW1) suggests that all the name alternatives that the group members can come up with could be collected over the following week by writing them on a piece of paper on the wall (lines 1–17; lines 3–17 not shown in the transcript).

Extract 4a

```
01 SW1:  mitä jos laitetaan sellanen (.) lappu
         what if we would put the kind of (.) paper

02       johonki tohon seinälle
         somewhere there on the wall

((lines 3-17 removed))

18 Kati: no o:nhan se hyvä jos niit on ninku (.)
         well it is certainly good if there are those (.)

19       seinäl nähtävissä niitä nimiehdotuksia ni,
         visible on the wall those name suggestions so,

20       (0.2) on siin sit ainaki sillee (.)
         (0.2) at least then they are there like (.)

21       vähä mie°ttiä° (1.0) #et oisko sit
         a bit to be thought about (1.0) that would it be

22       joku muu ku se äs tee# valme°nnus sitte°
         something else than the ST-couching then

23       (7.0)

24 SW1:  sä  ehdotat   että kysytään?
         SG2 suggest-2 CP   ask-PASS
         you suggest that we ask?

25       (1.0)

26 Kati: ↑n::iin on se hy[vä v]armaan nii.
         P        be it good  I.guess  P
         ↑ye:a:h it is go[od I] guess yea.

27 SW1:                 [nii,]
                        [yea,]
```

In response to SW1's proposal, a client, Kati, assesses the proposal in a positive way (lines 18–22), thus bringing the sequence a major step forward toward a decision. However, Kati's turn is followed by a long silence (line 23), after which the support worker reformulates Kati's positive stance toward the idea, inviting her to confirm it ("you suggest that we ask," line 24). After a one-second silence (line 25), Kati provides such confirmation ("ye:a:h it is good I guess yea," line 26), but her utterance involves signs of hesitance: a long stretch in the prosodic production of the particle *niin* "yeah" and the use of the epistemic adverb *varmaan* "I guess." Given the lack of substantial commitment to the proposed action, SW2 redirects the request for commitment to the entire group (line 28).

Extract 4b

28 SW2: mitä muut sanoo.
what do the others say.

29 (5.0)

30 Make: hiljasta.
silent.

31 SW1: hiljasta o(h)n heh näin o. ((laughter))
silent i(h)t is heh that's right.

32 (7.0)

33 SW2: **no ↑mä ehdotan kans sitä äänesty[s,**
P SG1 suggest-1 also it-PAR voting
well ↑I also suggest that votin [g

34 SW1: [↑mm,
[↑mm,

35 (1.0)

36 SW2: tai sitä ehdote- eh[dotus]asiaa.
or that voting- vot[ing t]hing.

37 SW1: [↑nii.]
[↑yea.]

38 SW2: mennäänks sillä.
shall we go with that.

39 SW1: ↑mennään sillä. haluuksä Kati tehä
↑let's go with that. do you Kati want to make

40 sellasen jonku lapun tuohon seinään.
some kind of paper on that wall.

After SW2's question, two long silences emerge (lines 29 & 32)—an awkward state of affairs that is also explicitly addressed in the conversation (lines 30–31). Finally, SW2—the colleague of the maker of the original proposal—announces her positive stance toward the proposed idea (lines 33 & 36). With the particle *kans* "also" (line 33), she casts her stance-taking as second to that of Kati, thus working toward constructing the emerging outcome of the sequence as a collective one. Thereafter, SW1 and SW2 together bring the decision-making process to completion by a series of displays of commitment (lines 38–39), which is followed by a request from SW1 to Kati to implement the decision ("do you Kati want to make some kind of paper on that wall," lines 39–40). Thus, even if one of the clients has taken a positive stance toward the support worker's proposal "in principle," the actual emergence of the decision is largely a result of the collaborative effort of the two support workers.

Conclusions

This chapter has described how support workers in mental health rehabilitation meetings at the Clubhouse seek to encourage the client members of the community to participate in making decisions about their communal life. While promoting client participation, the support workers also need to ascertain that at least some decisions get constructed during the meetings. As we have shown in our analysis, this combination of goals—promoting participation and constructing decisions—leads to a series of dilemmatic practices occurring at different points in the decision-making sequence. The support workers may treat a client's turn retrospectively as a proposal, even if the status of the client's turn as such is ambiguous. In the face of a lack of recipient uptake, the support workers may remind the clients about their epistemic access to the content of the proposal or pursue their agreement or commitment to the proposed plan. These practices involve the support workers carrying more responsibility over the unfolding of interaction and the emergence of decisions than the clients do.

As has been repeatedly argued in our analysis, the idea of support workers carrying a relatively large share of responsibility over the unfolding of interaction and the emergence of decisions compromises the genuine jointness of the decision-making outcome. Nonetheless, the support workers' conduct can be accounted for with reference to two general perspectives, which we will briefly attend to below.

First, the support workers' conduct can be accounted for with reference to the nature of social interactional practices as fundamentally *cooperative* (e.g., Tomasello, 2009). Thus, the unequal distribution of responsibility in interaction is not at all exceptional in human social life. Instead, it is common that a more skilled participant, on demand, takes an active role in solving problems of interaction (e.g., Goffman, 1955; Goodwin, 1995; Laakso, 2012). Such collaboration has been extensively studied in situations that involve asymmetry in the participants' communication skills, for example, in second-language interactions (Kurhila, 2006) or in conversations with participants with aphasia (Goodwin, 1995; Laakso, 2015) or hearing impairment (Scarinci, Worral, & Hickson, 2008). The findings from our data can thus also be accounted for with reference to the support workers simply compensating for the difficulties mental health clients have to participate in joint decision-making, In so doing, they helped to maintain the smooth unfolding of interaction and allowed for the emergence of at least some decisions during the meetings.

Second, the support workers' conduct can be understood from the perspective of pedagogy. Their practices reflect what Vehviläinen (2014) has referred to as a *supporting orientation* in counseling, in which the professional is active in maintaining both the participants' interaction and the client's involvement in it. From this perspective, the support workers' practices can also be conceptualized with reference to the notions of *scaffolding* (Snow, 1977) and *the zone of proximal development* (Vygotsky, 1978), when it is essential to treat the learners as somewhat more competent than they actually are. In mental health rehabilitation group meetings, this would entail the clients also participating in the kind of decision-making processes that they could not participate in independently—without the support workers' assistance (Vygotsky, 1978). Arguably, learning happens when the clients become socialized into the practices of the group and their developing joint decision-making skills become independent of the support workers' assistance (see John-Steiner & Mann, 1996). From this perspective, a specific challenge in the context of group meetings is generated by the differences of competence between group members and the changes of competence associated with the processes of illness recovery. In our data, such challenges might have been at stake, for example, in Extracts 4a and 4b, in which only one client participated in the decision-making, with the other clients remaining silent even in the face of long and awkward silences.

While there are ways to make sense of the support workers' conduct during the mental health rehabilitation group meetings at the Clubhouse, potential drawbacks of such conduct are also inevitable. As repeatedly pointed out in our analysis, one such drawback has to do with the opportunity to reject proposals in an easy and face-saving way. While an explicit rejection of a proposal can be a challenging conversational act to accomplish in any situation, such a rejection is even more difficult to produce in situations such as the ones analyzed in this chapter, when the proposer displays a lot of investment in his or her proposal by actively pursuing it in the face of a lack of recipient uptake. Sometimes there may be *two* support workers aligning with each other in advancing a proposal, which makes a rejection of a proposal an even more demanding action to produce. Another possible drawback has to do with the "meta-level" management of the joint decision-making interaction in the kinds of informal decision-making settings in which the decision-making agenda should be just as negotiable as the content of the decisions to be made. While the mere act of making a proposal entails a claim about its relevance for the group, the chance to respond to the proposal with silence is a way to display implicit resistance toward such a claim. This why the practices of promoting participation are inherently dilemmatic.

The practices to promote client participation are thus inevitably a matter of power and control, not only over the *content* of the decisions to be made, but also over *whether*, *when*, and *on what* decisions should be made in the first place. This inherently dilemmatic nature of promoting participation is worth keeping in mind especially in the high-stakes decision-making situations in which the genuine "jointness" of joint decision-making is of particular importance to the client's physical or mental well-being.

Acknowledgements This study (and the studies reported in Chapters 6, 8, 9, and 12) was funded by the Academy of Finland (Grant No. 307630) and the University of Helsinki.

References

Barry, M. J., & Edgman-Levitan, S. (2012). Shared decision making: The pinnacle of patient-centered care. *New England Journal of Medicine, 366*(9), 780–781.

Beitinger, R., Kissling, W., & Hamann, J. (2014). Trends and perspectives of shared decision-making in schizophrenia and related disorders. *Current Opinion in Psychiatry, 27*(3), 222–229.

Chamberlin, J. (1990). The ex-patients' movement: Where we've been and where we're going. *Journal of Mind and Behavior, 11*(3&4), 323–336.

Charles, C., Gafni, A., & Whelan, T. (1999). Decision-making in the physician-patient encounter: Revisiting the shared treatment decision-making model. *Social Science and Medicine, 49*(5), 651–692.

Davidson, L., O'Connell, M. J., Tondora, J., Lawless, M., & Evans, A. C. (2005). Recovery in serious mental illness: A new wine or just a new bottle? *Professional Psychology: Research and Practice, 36*(5), 480–487.

Drake, R. E., Deegan, P. E., & Rapp, C. (2010). The promise of shared decision making in mental health. *Psychiatric Rehabilitation Journal, 34*(1), 7–13.

Elstad, T. A., & Eide, A. H. (2009). User participation in community mental health services: Exploring the experiences of users and professionals. *Scandinavian Journal of Caring Science, 23*(4), 674–681.

Epstein, R. M., Franks, P., Fiscella, K., Cleveland, G. S., Meldrum, S. C., Kravitz, R., & Duberstein, P. R. (2005). Measuring patient-centred communication in patient-physician consultations: Theoretical and practical issues. *Social Science and Medicine, 61*(7), 1516–1528.

Ernst, M., & Paulus, M. P. (2005). Neurobiology of decision making: A selective review from a neurocognitive and clinical perspective. *Biological Psychiatry, 58*(8), 597–604.

Goffman, E. (1955). On face work: An analysis of ritual elements in social interaction. *Psychiatry: Journal for the Study of Interpersonal Processes, 18*(3), 213–231.

Goodwin, C. (1995). Co-constructing meaning in conversation with an aphasic man. *Research on Language and Social Interaction, 28*(3), 233–260.

Hänninen, E. (2012). *Choices for recovery: Community-based rehabilitation and the Clubhouse Model as means to mental health reforms*. Helsinki: National Institute for Health and Welfare.

Hänninen, E. (Ed.) (2016). *Mieleni minun tekevi: Mielenterveyskuntoutujien Klubitalot 20 vuotta Suomessa* [I would like to: Clubhouses for mental health rehabilitation 20 years in Finland]. Helsinki: Lönnberg.

Hickey, G., & Kipping, C. (1998). Exploring the concept of user involvement in mental health through a participation continuum. *Journal of Clinical Nursing, 7*(1), 83–88.

John-Steiner, V., & Mann, H. (1996). Sociocultural approaches to learning and development: A Vygotskian framework. *Educational Psychologist, 31*(3–4), 191–206.

Kurhila, S. (2006). *Second language interaction*. Amsterdam: Benjamins.

Laakso, M. (2012). Aphasia as an example of how a communication disorder affects interaction. In M. Egbert & A. Deppermann (Eds.), *Hearing Aids Communication* (pp. 138–145). Mannheim: Verlag für Gesprächsforschung.

Laakso, M. (2015). Collaborative participation in aphasic word searching: Comparison between significant others and speech and language therapists. *Aphasiology, 29*(3), 269–290.

Larquet, M., Coricelli, G., Opolczynski, G., & Thibaut, F. (2010). Impaired decision making in schizophrenia and orbitofrontal cortex lesion patients. *Schizophrenia Research, 116*(2), 266–273.

Niemi, J. (2010). Myönnyttelymuotti: Erimielisyyttä enteilevä samanmielisyyden konstruktio [Concession format: Construction of agreement anticipating disagreement]. *Virittäjä, 114*(2), 196–222.

Sacks, H., & Schegloff, E. A. (1973). Opening up closings. *Semiotica, 8*(4), 289–327.

Scarinci, N., Worrall, L., & Hickson, L. (2008). The effect of hearing impairment in older people on the spouse. *International Journal of Audiology, 47*(3), 141–151.

Schegloff, E. A. (2007). *Sequence organization in interaction: A primer in conversation analysis*. Cambridge: Cambridge University Press.

Sidnell, J. (2013). Basic conversation analytic method. In J. Sidnell & T. Stivers (Eds.), *The handbook of conversation analysis* (pp. 77–99). Chichester: Wiley-Blackwell.
Snow, C. E. (1977). The development of conversation between mothers and babies. *Journal of Child Language, 4*(1), 1–22.
Stevanovic, M. (2012). Establishing joint decisions in a dyad. *Discourse Studies, 14*(6), 779–803.
Stevanovic, M. (2015). Displays of uncertainty and proximal deontic claims: The case of proposal sequences. *Journal of Pragmatics, 78*, 84–97.
Stevanovic, M., & Peräkylä, A. (2012). Deontic authority in interaction: The right to announce, propose and decide. *Research on Language and Social Interaction, 45*(3), 297–321.
Tomasello, M. (2009). *Why we cooperate*. Cambridge, MA: MIT Press.
Treichler, E. B., & Spaulding, W. D. (2017). Beyond shared decision-making: Collaboration in the age of recovery from serious mental illness. *American Journal of Orthopsychiatry, 87*(5), 567–574.
Valkeapää, T., Lindholm, C., Tanaka, K., Weiste, E., & Stevanovic, M. (2019). Interaction, ideology, and practice in mental health rehabilitation. *Journal of Psychosocial Rehabilitation and Mental Health, 6*(1), 9–23.
Vehviläinen, S. (2014). *Ohjaustyön opas: Yhteistyössä kohti toimijuutta* [Guide for counselling work: In cooperation toward agency]. Helsinki: Gaudeamus.
Vygotsky, L. (1978). *Thought and language*. Cambridge, MA: MIT Press.

3

Attending to Parent and Child Rights to Make Medication Decisions During Pediatric Psychiatry Visits

Lisa Mikesell, F. Alethea Marti, Jennifer R. Guzmán, Michael McCreary, and Bonnie T. Zima

Fostering children's participation in their healthcare is increasingly recommended as good clinical practice (American Academy of Pediatrics, 2016). Children's participation has been linked to more accurate data gathering, cooperation with treatment, improved child safety, and heightened feelings of well-being (Alderson, Sutcliffe, & Curtis, 2006; De Winter, Baerveldt, & Kooistra, 2002; Runeson, Hallstrom, Elander, & Hermeren, 2002; Tiffenberg, Wood, Alonso, Tossuti, & Vincente, 2000; Vis, Standbu, Holten, & Thomas, 2011). With a growing orientation to

L. Mikesell (✉)
Department of Communication, Rutgers University,
New Brunswick, NJ, USA
e-mail: lisa.mikesell@rutgers.edu

Institute for Health, Health Care Policy and Aging Research
at Rutgers University, New Brunswick, NJ, USA

F. A. Marti · M. McCreary · B. T. Zima
Center for Health Services and Society,
University of California, Los Angeles, CA, USA
e-mail: fmarti@ucla.edu

C. Lindholm et al. (eds.), *Joint Decision Making in Mental Health*,
The Language of Mental Health, https://doi.org/10.1007/978-3-030-43531-8_3

children's rights and self-determination, supporting children's participation is also recommended on moral grounds (Oldfield & Fowler, 2004). Yet, despite these continued calls, research estimates that children's (aged 6–12) involvement accounts for between 3 and 14.2% of visits and most frequently occurs during social rather than instrumental talk (Coyne, 2008; Van Dolmen, 1998). Morever, when children are involved instrumentally in their care, it tends to be during history taking or data gathering and less often when treatment decisions are made (Cahill & Papageorgiou, 2007; see Coyne, 2008; Tates, Meeuwesen, Elbers, & Bensin, 2002; Wiering et al., 2016). Relatedly, interventions developed to improve shared decision-making in pediatrics predominantly target parents, not children (Wyatt et al., 2015). These findings suggest that, despite efforts to validate children's involvement in their care, including children—particularly in decision-making—remains challenging.

Such challenges may be heightened in interactions with children diagnosed with attention-deficit/hyperactivity disorder (ADHD) given characteristic symptoms of inattention, hyperactivity, and impulsivity (American Psychiatric Association, 2013). The use of stimulant medication in combination with behavioral therapy is the recommended treatment for children older than six years of age with an ADHD diagnosis (American Academic of Pediatrics, 2011). While stimulants have been found to reduce ADHD symptoms (e.g., improve focus, organizational skills) and

---

M. McCreary
e-mail: mmccreary@mednet.ucla.edu

J. R. Guzmán
Department of Anthropology,
State University of New York, Geneseo, NY, USA
e-mail: guzman@geneseo.edu

B. T. Zima
Department of Psychiatry and Biobehavioral Sciences,
University of California, Los Angeles, CA, USA
e-mail: bzima@mednet.ucla.edu

benefit children academically and socially, documented side effects include decreased appetite, sleep disorders, headaches, stomach pain, and irritability (Padhilla, Virtuoso, Tonin, Borba, & Pontarolo, 2018). While there have been considerable efforts to understand parental involvement in ADHD medication decisions, there has been less research exploring children's involvement (Honeycutt, Sleath, Bush, Campbell, & Tudor, 2005). Given the potential impact of stimulants on children's quality of life and everyday experience, how and when children influence stimulant decisions seems particularly worthwhile to explore.

Using video recordings of pediatric psychiatry consultations during medication titration for newly diagnosed children recently prescribed a stimulant, this chapter explores children's real-time participation in stimulant decisions, particularly how children's deontic rights—their rights to determine future actions (Stevanovic & Peräkylä, 2012)—are interactionally attended to and negotiated. During medication titration, pediatric psychiatrists monitor incremental dose increases of the prescribed stimulant to maximize benefits and minimize side effects (Brinkman et al., 2016). Accordingly, these consultations largely center on determining any changes in treatment after children trial a change in medication or dose. This environment thus presents an opportunity to carefully consider how children with documented behavioral concerns may come to participate in decisions about medications that impact their quality of life (McCabe, Rushton, Glover, Murray, & Keikin, 1996).

Treatment Recommendations and Child Participation

Conversation analytic research has described the interactional moment when medication decisions are made as part of the treatment recommendation (TR) phase of a clinic visit (see Heritage & Maynard, 2006). This work has focused on acute primary care visits where during the TR phase (see Robinson, 2003 on primary care activity phases) clinicians provide "instruction" to engage in some future action to benefit the patient (Byrne & Long, 1976). While TRs in primary care may include instructions for further testing or seeing a specialist, TRs during medication titration often entail recommendations to remain on the current medication, start/stop a medication, or make a dose adjustment. While clinicians' medical expertise may afford them epistemic rights to deliver TRs, research has shown that TRs are not unilateral actions; rather, they are treated as negotiable products of interaction and as normatively requiring patient acceptance. For instance, providers in general medicine and oncology have been found to seek patient acceptance of the TR (Costello & Roberts, 2001). When patients withhold acceptance, whether through passive (e.g., remaining silent) or active (e.g., asking questions) resistance, providers have been shown to pursue acceptance by providing accounts for their TRs or modifying them (Costello & Roberts, 2001; Koenig, 2011; Parry, 2009; Stivers, 2005a, 2005b, 2006, 2007). Accordingly, Koenig (2011) argues that such resistance practices constitute resources for patients to secure TRs that are more in line with their expectations.

In pediatric acute care, studies show that physicians often pursue TR acceptance from parents and it is parents' resistance to TRs that influence TR delivery (Stivers, 2005a, 2005b, 2006). As Stivers (2005a) notes, contrary to previous work claiming that patient/parent participation in decision-making is dependent on clinicians' explicit invitations, parent participation, even when not invited, influences the decisions ultimately made. What role children play, if any, in negotiating TRs has been less explored.

Several factors influence how children come to participate in healthcare encounters including children's age and maturity (Irwin & Johnson, 2005; Pantell, Stewart, Dias, Wells, & Ross, 1982); physician experience and specialty (Honeycutt et al., 2005; Irwin & Johnson, 2005); children's gender, race, and socioeconomic status (Stivers & Majid, 2007); and parental presence (Ringnér, Öster, Björk, & Graneheim, 2012; Tates & Meeuwesen, 2000). Research also shows that children are not always forthcoming or cogent in their responses (Stivers, 2001; see Stivers, Sidnell, & Bergen, 2018) and that clinicians may perceive children's involvement as problematic (Runseon, Enskär, Elander, & Hermerén, 2001), both of which may influence rates of child participation. Additionally, triadic healthcare contexts constitute complex communication environments (Dalton, 2003; Irwin & Johnson, 2005) with interactional factors contributing to how children participate. For instance, pediatricians can select the parent or child as recipients of their turns, or address both parent and child (e.g., by addressing turns to "you guys") leaving the parent and child to work out who will respond. Speaker selection has consequences for participation by determining, for example, which party will present the child's problem (Stivers, 2001). Pediatricians have been found to select parents more often than children (60% vs. 37%) as recipients to questions, perhaps because parents respond more frequently to questions that select them than do children (93% vs. 65%) (Stivers & Majid, 2007; see also Tates & Meeuwesen, 2001). Moreover, even when children are selected, parents may speak on their behalf (Aronsson & Rundstrom, 1988; Nova, Vegni, & Moja, 2005), further limiting children's participation.

Importantly, mitigating such challenges may be possible. Stivers' (2012) identifies communication practices that contribute to clinicians' success in securing responses from children: relying on polar (yes–no) question designs, which children more readily answer (vs. Wh-questions; see Irwin & Johnson, 2005), and gazing at children when delivering questions. Cahill and Papageorgiou (2007) similarly found that directing gaze at children and addressing them by name reduced caregivers' attempts to speak for children. While observational studies point to a number of factors influencing children's participation across the entire healthcare visit, how children are involved specifically in the task of making medication decisions and how their involvement might be supported is less evident (Coyne, 2008).

Research Questions

We were guided by the overarching question of how children's deontic rights to make decisions during medication titration for ADHD were attended to. We asked:

1. What practices do clinicians draw on during the TR phase to invite or encourage children to participate in medication decisions?
2. Do children volunteer medication preferences, positioning themselves as decision makers, and how does such participation shape clinicians' TR deliveries?

Data and Method

The data were collected as part of a pilot study examining the implementation of an mHealth web interface to improve medication titration (Mikesell, Marti, Guzman, McCreary, & Zima, 2018). The pilot data were collected in two phases (January 2014–November 2016; August 2017–October 2018), involving 14 clinicians at two community mental health clinics serving South Los Angeles and North Compton, California in the United States. Following an initial visit (not recorded) in which an ADHD diagnosis was made and a stimulant prescribed, families returned for follow-up visits to discuss the medication's effects and possible adjustments to the type of medication or dose.

Families were eligible to participate if (1) the parent's primary language was English; (2) the child was between 5 and 11 years old; and (3) the child had received a clinical diagnosis of ADHD and a first-time stimulant medication prescription. Families were excluded from participating if the child had (1) any chronic medical condition that required ongoing medication management; (2) a prior prescription of psychotropic medication; and (3) moderate–severe development delays, intellectual disability, or autism.

In total, 18 families participated. Two children never began medication because of diagnostic uncertainty so were omitted from the current analysis. Each family agreed to be recorded for three follow-up visits. However, only 14 families recorded three consecutive visits; one family recorded only the second follow-up visit and one family recorded the first two visits only. Thus, the data set includes 16 English-speaking families participating in 45 video-recorded follow-up visits with 14 clinicians, totaling 24.4 hours of data. Visit length ranged between 14.5 and 63.1 minutes ($M = 32.9$; SD = 12.1). Six of the 16 (37.5%) children participated during the TR phase across 10 of the 45 (22.2%) visits involving five (35.7%) different clinicians.

To examine how children participate in medication decisions, for each visit we identified the clinician's TR or initiation of the treatment discussion and its recipient—whether it was designed for the parent (e.g., via eye gaze, by referring to the child in the third person), for the child (e.g., via eye gaze, hearably child-directed intonation, address terms), or whether the recipient was ambiguous such that a single intended recipient was unclear (e.g., addressing a question to "you guys"). We examined all TRs demonstrably delivered to children and to both parent and child to examine if and how children responded to them. We also catalogued all occasions when children volunteered a treatment preference during any phase of the visit and occasions when clinicians solicited children's preferences for medication (parents never sought children's preferences) during the TR phase.

Inviting Children to Comment on a Parent-Accepted TR

In most visits (93.3%, $n = 42$), clinicians initiated medication discussions with parents or delivered the TR to parents, thereby treating parents as the primary decision makers. For example, in Extract 1, the clinician, orienting to the mother's earlier reported concern that the increase in dose has caused a side effect, recommends keeping the child on the higher (27 mg) dose.

Extract 1

```
01 DOC: I think it's fine to keep him at twenty seven.=I
02      don't think you need to go back to the eightee:n.
03 MOM: Okay.
```

Clinicians most often sought children's perspective of a treatment after it had already been agreed to by the parent. That is, children were asked to provide their perspective on medication decisions that were effectively already made, revealing how clinicians attended to parents' deontic authority while acknowledging children's agency to comment on parents' decisions. In Extract 2, this invitation immediately follows the treatment discussion with the parent and occurs as a simple adjacency pair (Schegloff, 2007) involving two turns: the provider produces a first turn seeking the child's assessment of the parent-accepted TR followed by the child's positive assessment, which is treated as sequence closure.

Extract 2

```
01 MOM: Yes:.=
02 CHI: =£N(h)o(h)o(h):.£
03 DOC: Why don't we:- we'll leave it at this do:se until
04      the next time we see each other:,
05 MOM: Okay.
((lines 06-21 omitted))
22 DOC: We could even do that before we see each other: maybe
23      give it another couple wee:ks and see: an' then if
24      you feel like you would like to move it a little
25      later before we see each other, ask the school to do
26      it.=If they need a note from me to do it, just call
27      me and I can always fax something over to them.
28 MOM: Okay.
29 DOC: Okay? |How does that sou:nd.
30 doc         | ((shifts gaze to CHI))
31 CHI: Good.
32 DOC: Okay.
33 DOC: When do you get your first progress report?=Do
34      you know?
```

This child (age 8) was recently put on an additional 5 mg of stimulant. The clinician's initial TR presents mom two options with a clearly marked preference (Toerien, Shaw, & Reuber, 2013), which the mother accepts (not shown). After a talk with the child about helping mom at home (lines 1–2), the clinician redelivers the TR to mom (lines 3–4), which the mom again accepts (line 5). Following a discussion about adjusting the timing of the afternoon dose to address mom's reported difficulties after school (lines 22–28), the clinician seeks the child's perspective on the treatment plan as she and mom have just discussed (referenced by indexical "that"), directing her gaze toward the child when she asks: *How does that s_ou:nd.* (lines 29–30).

The Wh-question design provides leeway for the child to convey her independent assessment, particularly in comparison to polar questions that embed a grammatical preference and may exert interactional pressure to agree (Heritage, 2010; see Extract 4, line 43): for example, *Does that sound alright?* or *Is that okay (with you)?* are grammatically designed for "yes" responses (Boyd & Heritage, 2006). Although the question here does not convey such a preference, its "how" format imposes constraints on the type of expected response, namely, a qualitative assessment (e.g., "good," "okay"). Such constraints may serve as resources for children to more readily produce a normative response (see Stivers, 2001, 2012; compare the Wh-question design in Extract 4, line 23). Here the child responds promptly with "good" (line 30) indicating a positive stance toward and thus agreement with mom's treatment decision. Having secured the mother's acceptance of the TR and the child's agreement with mom's decision (line 31), the TR phase comes to a close (line 32) and the clinician shifts to a new activity (lines 33–34).

The clinician in Extract 3 similarly employs a "how"-formatted question to elicit the child's assessment of a parent-accepted TR. Notably, this extract also reveals how children's resistance practices can shape the TR that is ultimately delivered and may also assist in creating the interactional environment that occasions clinicians to invite children's assessments.

Extract 3

```
01 DOC: .hh Welm- it sounds like the twenty-seven is
02      helpi:ng,
03      (.)
04 chi  (0.2) ((head|shake, looks at DOC))
05 DOC:             |We don't kno::w if it's causing a
06 doc              |((gazes to MOM))
07 DOC: heada:che, w'l-but let's keep it at the twenty-
08      seven for no:w and see:.
09 MOM: Okay.
10 DOC: |(An' it's- |ne-) o k a:: y ?|
11 doc  |            |((looks at CHI)) |
12 chi  | ((l o o k i n g  d o w n )) |((looks at DOC))
13 DOC: Elijah, how do you feel about tha:t.
14 CHI: M:: ((nods))
15 DOC: >Ho-<You feel okay with tha:t?
16 CHI: ((nods))
17      (0.2)
18 DOC: Okay.
```

Following the clinician's positive summary of the medication's effectiveness to the mother (lines 1–2), the child (age 11) shakes his head in disagreement (line 4). In the face of disagreement, the clinician, looking to mom (line 6), continues her summary acknowledging the child's earlier reported headache while also posing doubt that the medication is the cause (lines 5, 7). The clinician is still gazing at the mother when she produces her TR (lines 7–8; *let's keep it at the twenty-seven for no:w and see:.*), which mom readily accepts (line 9).

Following mom's acceptance, the clinician looks to the child who is looking down and mobilizes a response (line 10) with rising intoned *oka:::y?*, which she lengthens until she secures the child's gaze (line 12). Having garnered his attention, she elicits his perspective about the decision mom has agreed to with a "how" question similar to Extract 2: *Elijah, how do yo̲u feel about tha:t.* Although the question seeks the child's assessment of the decision, the child nods in response, treating the question as a polar question. The nod's ill-fittedness to the question design only opaquely conveys a positive stance, which may occasion the clinician's subsequent inquiry (line 15). In her follow-up, she abandons the "how" question format to produce a polar question whose grammatical preference aligns with the child's previous "yes" response (*Ho- you feel oka̲y with tha:t?*). The child nods again, officially confirming the parent-accepted TR, which brings the TR phase to a close (line 18).

Extract 4 shows a clinician who elicits the child's independent perspective (rather than assessment) of a parent-accepted TR with a "what"-formatted Wh-question (rather than a "how"-formatted question). The child (age 8) displays difficultly responding to this open-ended question and the mother and clinician pursue a response, treating the child's perspective as required for closing the TR phase.

Extract 4

```
01 DOC: Um so y'know it's really: eh-e sounds like she's
02      doing quite we:ll.
03 mom  ((nods))
04 DOC: There maybe is some fine tuning to happen in the
05      later part of the da:y. We can wait if you want to
06      get some feedback from the adults who were working
07      with her in the later part of the da::y, or we can
08      even just go ahead and add it now.<I don't think it
09      would hurt at all. She's on a- a small dose.=Ten is-
10      ten is sma:ll.
11 MOM: Yea.
((lines 12-21 omitted; talk about school administering dose))
22 DOC: I can certainly write something on a letter.
23 DOC: .hh Okay well what do you think Sammy.
24      (0.5)
25 DOC: I'm interested if you think that having a little
26      bit later in the day could be helpful.
27 chi  (4.5) ((playing with tooth))
28 mom  ((taps child))
29 MOM: [Did you understand] what she said?
30 DOC: [(                 )
31 chi  ((headshake))
32 DOC: heh heh heh .hhh So: it sounds like the medication
33      is helping you- quite a bit. During the school day.
34      And maybe it's wearing off kind of later in the
35      da::y?
36      (0.3)
37 DOC: So we can add a little bit (0.2) later in the day
38      to help you with like your after-school program
39      ti::me, or whatever later:: classes you have,
40      subjects.
41      (0.2)
42 DOC: Nkay?
43 DOC: .hh Do you think that you would wanna try tha:t?
44 chi  ((nods))
45 DOC: Okay.
```

The clinician presents two treatment options for mom to consider (lines 4–10; see Landmark, Gulbrandsen, & Svennevig, 2015; Toerien, Shaw, Duncan, & Reuber, 2011), noting that the second option of adding a dose in the afternoon requires the school to dispense it. Mom implies a preference for this option when she reports that she has already discussed this with the school (not shown). With a shift implicative *Okay* (line 23; Beach, 1995), the clinician turns to the child and solicits her perspective on the just prior treatment discussion. In the prior extracts, the "how"-formatted questions enabled children to merely *claim* understanding of the TR they were assessing and thus potentially obscure any difficulty genuinely understanding the TR. Here, the question—*Well what do you think Sammy.*—encourages the child to *demonstrate* understanding of the TR (Sacks, 1992).

The child may face several challenges responding. Given that the TR is discussed across an extended sequence with more than one treatment option, it may be unclear which option she is being asked to consider. However, when the child delays responding (line 24), the doctor clarifies that she is inquiring specifically about the second option for which mom has indicated a preference (i.e., *having a little bit later in the day*; lines 25–26); this clarification does not seem to resolve the trouble (lines 27–31). The clinician further explains the treatment option (lines 32–40), which also receives no uptake from the child (lines 36, 41). The clinician then works to mobilize a response (line 42) and produces a "yes"-preferring polar question to secure the child's explicit agreement with mom's implied preference (line 43). This shift to a polar question provides stronger design constraints limiting the child's response to "yes" or "no" (Stivers, 2012). While this question design minimizes the opportunity for the child to voice her independent perspective on the TR that the initial Wh-question sought, it allows the child to claim rather than demonstrate understanding (Sacks, 1992) of the TR, perhaps enabling her to respond more readily. The child nods (line 44), indicating her acceptance of the TR, which brings sequence closure (line 45).

In sum, inviting children's participation during the TR phase was infrequent and such invitations prioritized parents' deontic authority by seeking parent's decisions before inviting children to participate. At the same time, when clinicians invited children's perspectives on the medication decision, they did so with open-ended questions to invite children's independent assessments or perspectives and their responses were treated as required for bringing the TR sequence to closure.

Delivering TRs to Children

On two occasions, clinicians delivered the TR directly to the child. Notably, in both cases, clinicians' TR deliveries were responsive to interactional contingencies (see also Extract 7). For instance, Extract 5 shows that delivering the TR to the child may not principally work to secure the child's acceptance, but rather to pull his attention away from a competing discussion, allowing the clinician to return to the institutional business at hand.

Extract 5

```
01 DOC: Okay. ↑We:[ll
02 CHI:           [Can we go to the park today?
03      (0.3)
04 doc  | ((gazing at child))
05 DOC: |I thi[nk u:m
06 AUN:         [(m::) w:e'll see.
07 CHI: Tomorrow.
08 DOC: Jayvo|n I
09 aun        |((shifts gaze to DOC))
10 DOC: [↑think-
11 CHI: [cause we have school (        ).
12 DOC: I think maybe we should give you: |a slightly
13 chi                                    |((gazes to DOC))
14 DOC: higher dose of the medici:ne that u:m maybe just
15      stick with the short acting o:ne since the lo:ng
16      acting one you seem to have some problems with.
17 AUN: Yea it make him hyper.
```

As the clinician begins to move from the prior activity of data gathering to the TR phase with a shift implicative "okay" (line 1), the child (age 7) asks his aunt to go to the park (line 2). After a gap, the clinician and aunt compete for the floor (lines 5–6) and the aunt's inconclusive *we'll see* response to the child's request launches negotiations (line 7). In the midst of this derailment of the institutional agenda, the clinician addresses the child by name (line 8) and, upon hearable completion of his turn (line 11), she delivers the TR directly to him. This works to secure the attention of both the aunt (line 9) and eventually the child (line 13) and thus refocus the talk on the institutional task of delivering the TR (lines 12, 14–16). While delivering the TR to the child may provide the opportunity for the child to accept/reject it, in this case, it appears to be deployed to bring attention back to the institutional agenda that the child's request has derailed. Notably, even though the TR is addressed to the child, the clinician shifts gaze between the child and aunt during its delivery, and it is the aunt who responds (line 17).

Extract 6 shows the complexity of the triadic context in shaping how children may come to respond to the TR *before* the parent. As in the majority of cases, the TR here is first delivered to the parent. When the mother withholds her response (Stivers, 2005a), the clinician works to mobilize one from both the mother and child when she solicits a response from "you guys" (Lerner, 2003; Stivers, 2001). The child (age 8) seizes the opportunity to respond and immediately rejects the TR. However, the child's initial rejection receives no verbal uptake, and acceptance of the TR is ultimately pursued from the mother.

Extract 6

```
01 DOC: O:kay. .hh So I was talking t- to my team a little
02      bit and this is very |good. I- it is very good. I
03 doc                       |((gazes at MOM))
04      don't- The one thing I would like to do though is
05      try a higher |do:se .hh just to make sure we're not
06 mom:              |((nodding))
07 DOC: missing (0.3) if she's gonna do better at a higher
08      dose.
09      (0.4)
10 DOC: Would you guys wanna try that? Just a twenty-se-
11      trying the twenty seven?=
12 CHI: =NO.
13      (0.4)
14 CHI: Yes?=
15 DOC: =°heh heh heh [heh°
16 CHI:               [No yes, mo::m.
17      (0.2)
18 CHI: °No?=
19 doc  |((shifts gaze to MOM))
20 MOM: |=huh [huh huh huh
21 DOC:       [heh he
22 DOC: Well I- the reason I would wanna try it is just
23      to see. So we would try the twenty seve:n and you
24      say- if teacher says wow she's doing so much better
25      eve:n, .hhh and there's not any side effects then
26      we say oka:y maybe we should try this dose. 'Cause
27      um if you're saying no:: there's not improvement
28      and there's more side effects? we would go back
29      down. To the other one. We would [know in a couple
30 MOM:                                  [(mm)
31 DOC: of days.
32 DOC: I think that would be the smart thing to try.
33 MOM: °Okay.
```

The clinician first delivers the TR to *try a higher do:se* to the mom (via gaze, line 3; and referencing the child in the third person, line 7), who nods during the TR delivery (line 6) but does not verbally accept the TR (line 9). In the face of such weak resistance (Koenig, 2011; Stivers, 2005a), the clinician works to secure an acceptance: *Would you guys wanna try that?* (lines 10–11). Asking about desires to "try" a medication implicates the child, and she mobilizes a response from *you guys* (leaving the intended recipient ambiguous). The child latches her turn to the clinician's question and overtly and emphatically (with audible stress) rejects the TR (line 12). Upon no uptake of the child's rejection (line 13), the child backs down, modifying her initial rejection that was delivered with conviction to a tentatively produced (i.e., rising intoned) acceptance (lines 14). The clinician laughs in the face of the child's contradictory responses, but otherwise the child receives no verbal acknowledgment. The child waffles again, this time soliciting mom's assistance (line 16), which does not immediately come (line 17), and then the child revises her response a fourth time (line 18), producing her initial rejection but delivering it much less decisively with rising intonation and slightly lowered volume.

In response to the child's flip-flopping stances, both the mother (line 20) and clinician (line 21) laugh. While treating the child's responses as laughable and nonserious may in effect minimize her contributions, her uncertain rejection of the TR nevertheless prompts the clinician to offer an account for her recommendation to try a higher dose, making her clinical reasoning more transparent. Notably, the account is delivered to the mother (via gaze; line 19) (lines 22–31, 32) who is the party to accept the TR (line 33). Taken together, Extracts 5 and 6 illustrate participants' normative orientations to parents as the primary decision makers by detailing the "special" circumstances in which TRs are delivered to children. Additionally, even though children may be structurally afforded the opportunity to accept/reject the TR, acceptance is ultimately pursued from the parent.

When Children Volunteer Treatment Preferences

Although rare, children also volunteered treatment preferences, positioning *themselves* as the primary decision makers and thereby exerting "pressure" on clinicians to, in turn, treat them as having deontic rights to make decisions. Extract 7 shows one of two children, both age 11, who volunteered medication preferences and the only child to voice their preference *before* the TR was delivered (i.e., his preference is not responsive to a TR).

Extract 7

```
01 DOC: She gave something to the:m.
02      (0.3)
03 DOC: So it looks like she sai:::d
04 doc  (4.1) ((looking at computer))
05 CHI: I don't think you should move it u:p.
06      (0.2)
07 CHI: My medication.
08 doc  (0.9) ((looking at computer))
09 DOC: Okay hold on one second. So she was saying (1.1) she
10      sa::w (0.8) Did he- did he forget a dose? Maybe last
11      wee:k? ((lines 12-41 omitted))
42      ((DOC returns to room, sits down))
43 DOC: Okay Elija:h, so we:- I was talking with my boss, an'
44      (0.4) I know that you don't want to add another
45      medication::n? so what we will do: is we will
46      increase your medication by a tiny bit. .hh usually
47      I go up to thirty-si:x? But I'm just going to go up
48      a little bit to twenty-seven.
49 CHI: I don't wanna do tha:t.=
50 DOC: =Just a little bit jus' to see if that helps your
51      symptoms during the day.
```

Early in the visit, while the clinician is looking to see what the child's teacher reported (lines 1, 3), the child takes advantage of the silence (line 4) to voice his preference for not raising the dose (lines 5, 7). This occurs well before the TR phase when the clinician is attending to a distinctly different institutional activity and his contribution gets put on hold (line 9; see O'Reilly, 2006).

In volunteering his preference, the child demonstrates his understanding of the aims of medication titration and positions himself as having deontic rights to influence the decision. Later, when the TR phase is launched, the clinician follows suit, and rather than delivering the TR to the parent (who is present), she delivers it directly to him to accept/reject (lines 43–48). After addressing the child by name (line 43), she implicates her "boss" as part of the decision-making process diffusing responsibility for the TR (line 43), acknowledges the child's earlier stated preferences to not *add another medication* (lines 44–45), and then *pronounces* (see Stivers et al., 2017) the TR (lines 45–46). While pronouncement formats deliver the TR authoritatively, treating it as nonnegotiable (Stivers et al., 2017), the clinician accounts for her TR (cf. Peräkylä, 1998 regarding how clinicians balance authority/accountability during diagnosis), which acknowledges the child's earlier stated preferences. She explicates what she "usually" does (lines 46–48), implying that she is going against what is typical *because of* the child's preferences, a move that both treats her TR as an accountable matter and works to (unsuccessfully; line 49) ward off potential resistance from the child whose stated preferences contrast with her recommendation (see Bolden & Angell, 2017). On the one hand, the child, who positioned himself as the decision maker, is subsequently provided the first opportunity to reject/accept the TR and presented an account for the TR that is demonstrably attentive to his earlier expressed preferences. On the other hand, the clinician designs the TR as effectively decided by her and her team and thus not available for negotiation. As in many of the cases shown, this clinician attends to the child's agency to participate in the decision-making *process* but ultimately does not treat him as having the deontic authority to make the decision.

Discussion

The frameworks of patient-centered care and shared decision-making support a redistribution of deontic rights to foster patient autonomy (Sandman & Munthe, 2009). However, when the patient is a child accompanied by a parent, attending to the patient's deontic rights to make decisions may be complicated because of common understandings that "parents are the key decision makers regarding their child's health care" (Charach, Skyba, Cook, & Antle, 2006, p. 75). Physicians thus face significant pressures when having to engage a child patient and a parent (Tannen & Wallat, 1986, 1987). Although children's experiences with a medication are key to treatment decisions during medication titration, and thus call on clinicians to recognize children's treatment preferences, clinicians may also be sensitive to not challenge parents' deontic authority (Cahill & Papageorgiou, 2007).

Our findings seem to reflect these pressures clinicians are facing. Children's involvement during the TR phase when medication decisions are made was infrequent. Clinicians overwhelmingly initiated medication discussions with and delivered medication recommendations to parents, thus orienting to parents' deontic authority as decision makers. Moreover, the TR was delivered to children on only two occasions and was responsive to special interactional contingencies, further suggesting that treating children as having the primary rights to decide is rather exceptional. When clinicians invited children to participate in the medication decision, they notably balanced attention to parents' deontic authority by seeking children's assessments or perspectives of a TR that was already accepted by the parent. That is, clinicians attended to parents' commonly accepted status as the primary decision maker, while simultaneously recognizing children's agency to independently comment on the parent's decision. Thus, while clinicians worked to attend to both parents' and children's deontic rights to make medication decisions, they prioritized those of parents.

Given that children are rarely positioned as direct recipients of TRs, the same interactional resources afforded to parents to participate in the TR phase (i.e., passive and active resistance *in response to* TRs; see Koenig, 2011; Stivers, 2005a) may be more limited for children, requiring children to find alternative methods to assert their own deontic rights. Children's resistance, however, was also rare, and only two children volunteered medication preferences, suggesting that overall children also enacted a subordinate position to adults when it came to making treatment decisions. Given children's lack of initiation along with the infrequency with which TRs are delivered to them, children's inclusion in treatment decisions seems to require explicit support from adults, unlike parents who may influence treatment decisions even without clinician invitation (Stivers, 2005a). Importantly, our findings illustrate how some clinicians opted to provide this support.

Although parents' deontic authority was prioritized, children's deontic rights were attended to in the question designs clinicians relied on to invite children's participation; clinicians employed "how"-formatted Wh-questions to elicit children's assessments of the TR (*How does that sound.*) or "what"-formatted Wh-questions to invite children's perspectives on the TR (*Well what do you think*). They generally refrained from employing polar questions, which "by their very nature, present a hypothesis or candidate version of a state of affairs for confirmation" (Heritage, 2011, p. 340). In other words, clinicians typically invited children to do more than (dis)confirm a parent's decision by designing questions that enabled children to *independently* assess or comment on the parent-accepted TR. Although children have been found to more readily respond to polar questions (Stivers, 2012), clinicians seemed to reserve polar questions for pursuing responses after children showed difficulty answering clinicians' initial open invitations. Examining cases when children showed such difficulties also points to a possible communication mechanism underlying children's ability to respond more readily to polar questions: the confirmatory (yes/no) responses polar questions make relevant may enable children to merely claim rather than demonstrate understanding of the information being solicited (Sacks, 1992), rendering polar questions less demanding. Thus, although Wh-questions requiring demonstrations of understanding may provide children the freedom to more independently contribute to medication decisions, question designs imposing stricter constraints on children's responses are more likely to receive them. This tradeoff may present a practical problem for clinicians regarding whether to question children to receive a genuine response (i.e., an independent perspective in response to a Wh-question) or receive a response at all (i.e., confirmation to a polar question that may mask misunderstanding). This paradox essentially places the clinician in the position of determining whether to pose questions to constrain the response options and thereby enable children to participate normatively, or pose questions without constraints that enable children to contribute more substantially but which may in actuality be too demanding for some children to cope with.

In addition, when children were invited to participate, clinicians did not treat children's perspectives as optional, further displaying the importance of children's acceptance of the treatment decision. Clinicians pursued responses when children delayed them or displayed difficulties responding before moving to sequence closure. That is, they did not orient to children's trouble responding as reason to move on to other activities but rather held children accountable for responding. Notably, holding children accountable for responding was not inevitable to all questions in other activity phases of the consultation; for instance, there were times when clinicians let children's nonresponsiveness pass, suggesting that, once pursued, getting children's agreement with the TR "on record" was particularly important for closing the TR phase.

This study examined ADHD medication titration consultations in two clinics from one geographic location, thus limiting generalizability. The small number of cases in which children were involved in medication decisions and the lack of outcome measures reported similarly limits understanding of the potential range of clinicians' practices and their comparative effectiveness for involving children in ADHD medication decisions. Nevertheless, it seems clear that parents are afforded primary deontic rights to make decisions, even in this chronic care context when children's treatment preferences may be particularly important for addressing quality of life concerns. Although children in other health contexts have also been found to participate infrequently, these data render it difficult to determine whether the frequency or nature of clinicians' invitations were associated with children's ADHD diagnosis or merely their developmental status as children. Additionally, while children who participated during the TR phase tended to be older (than 7 years), the data did not allow for a systematic examination of the role of exogenous or demographic factors and how they differentially contributed to children's participation.

Lastly, this study may be limited by its exclusive focus on the TR phase. Children were routinely asked to share their medication experiences and more readily volunteered information during the data-gathering phase of these consultations (Mikesell, Marti, Guzman, McCreary, & Zima, 2017). Similar to adult patients, children's participation during these visits seems to vary across activities of the consultation (Cahill & Papageorgiou, 2007; see ten Have, 1991). Thus, our findings do not suggest that children's participation is equally limited across the entire visit. Regarding acute primary care visits, Robinson (2003) argues that the overarching project being oriented to for new medical problems is finding a solution to the problem, and that the other activity phases in primary care (e.g., data gathering, diagnosis) function to progress toward treatment. He suggests that, as a consequence, the overall structural organization of clinic activities exerts "pressure" on patient participation in systematic ways. Because this chapter does not detail the overall structural organization of medication titration visits, its relationship to child (and parent) participation was not adequately considered, and it may be that children's participation during other activities (e.g., data gathering) is treated as progressing toward treatment and thus contributing to treatment decisions. Nevertheless, we aimed to explore how children were specifically involved when ADHD medication decisions are made. According to our findings, some clinicians treat children as having limited deontic rights; while they orient to parents' decision-making authority, they recognize children's agency to comment on parents' decisions but do not generally recognize children's authority to make medication decisions themselves.

References

Alderson, P., Sutcliffe, K., & Curtis, K. (2006). Children as partners in their medical care. *Archives of Disease in Childhood, 91*, 300–303.

American Academic of Pediatrics. (2011). ADHD: Clinical practice guideline for the diagnosis, evaluation, and treatment of attention-deficit/hyperactivity disorder in children and adolescents. *Pediatrics, 128*(5), 1007–1022.

American Academy of Pediatrics. (2016). Informed consent in decision-making in pediatric practice. *Pediatrics, 138*(2), e20161484.

American Psychiatric Association. (2013). *Diagnostic and statistical manual of mental disorders* (5th ed.). Arlington, VA.

Aronsson, K., & Rundström, B. (1988). Child discourse and parental control in pediatric consultations. *Text, 8*, 159–184.

Beach, W. A. (1995). Conversation analysis: 'Okay' as a clue for understanding consequentiality. In S. J. Sigman (Ed.), *The consequentiality of communication* (pp. 121–161). Hillsdale, NJ: Lawrence Erlbaum.

Bolden, G. B., & Angell, B. (2017). The organization of the treatment recommendation phase in routine psychiatric visits. *Research on Language and Social Interaction, 50*(2), 151–170.

Boyd, E., & Heritage, J. (2006). Taking the patient's medical history: Questioning during comprehensive history taking. In J. Heritage & D. Maynard (Eds.), *Communication in medical care: Interactions between primary care physicians and patients* (pp. 151–184). New York: Cambridge University Press.

Brinkman, W. B., Baum, R., Kelleher, K. J., Peugh, J., Gardner, W., Lichtenstein, P., … Epstein, J. N. (2016). Relationship between attention-deficit/hyperactivity disorder care and medication continuity. *Journal of the American Academic of Child & Adolescent Psychiatry, 55*(4), 289–294.

Byrne, P. S., & Long, B. E. L. (1976). *Doctors talking to patients*. London: Her Majesty's Stationery Office.

Cahill, P., & Papageorgiou, A. (2007). Video analysis of paediatric consultations in primary care. *British Journal of General Practice, 57*(544), 866–871.

Charach, A., Skyba, A., Cook, L., & Antle, B. J. (2006). Using stimulant medication for children with ADHD: What do parents say? *Journal of Canadian Academic Child and Adolescent Psychiatry, 15*(2), 75–83.

Costello, B. A., & Roberts, F. (2001). Medical recommendations as joint social practice. *Health Communication, 13*(3), 241–260.

Coyne, I. (2008). Children's participation in consultations and decision-making in health service level: A review of the literature. *International Journal of Nursing Studies, 45*(11), 1682–1689.

Coyne, I., Mathuna, D., Gibson, F., Shields, L., Leclercq, E., & Sheaf, G. (2016). Interventions for promoting participation in shared decision-making for children with cancer. *Cochrane Database of Systematic Reviews, 11,* 1–31.

Dalton, J. M. (2003). Development and testing of the theory of collaborative decision-making in nursing practice for triads. *Journal of Advanced Nursing, 41*(1), 22–33.

De Winter, M., Baerveldt, C., & Kooistra, J. (2002). Enabling children: Participation as a new perspective on child-health promotion. *Child Care Health and Development, 28,* 109–116.

Heritage, J. (2010). Questioning in medicine. In A. F. Freed & S. Ehrlich (Eds.), *'Why do you ask?' The function of questions in institutional discourse* (pp. 43–68). Oxford: Oxford University Press.

Heritage, J. (2011). The interaction order and clinical practice: Some observations on dysfunctions and action steps. *Patient Education and Counseling, 84*(3), 338–343.

Heritage, J., & Maynard, D. (Eds.). (2006). *Communication in medical care: Interaction between physicians and patients.* Cambridge: Cambridge University Press.

Honeycutt, C., Sleath, B., Bush, P. J., Campbell, W., & Tudor, G. (2005). Physician use of a participatory decision-making style with children with ADHD and their parents. *Patient Education and Counseling, 57*(3), 327–332.

Irwin, L. G., & Johnson, J. (2005). Interviewing young children: Explicating our practice and dilemmas. *Qualitative Health Research, 15*(6), 821–831.

Koenig, J. C. (2011). Patient resistance as agency in treatment decisions. *Social Science and Medicine, 72*(7), 1105–1114.

Landmark, A. M. D., Gulbrandsen, P., & Svennevig, J. (2015). Whose decision? Negotiating epistemic and deontic rights in medical treatment decisions. *Journal of Pragmatics, 78*, 54–69.

Lerner, G. (2003). Selecting next speaker: The context-sensitive operation of a context-free organization. *Language in Society, 32*(3), 177–201.

McCabe, M. A., Rushton, C., Glover, J., Murray, M., & Leikin, S. (1996). Implications of the Patient Self Determination Act: Guidelines for involving adolescents in health care decision making. *Journal of Adolescent Health, 19*(5), 319–324.

Mikesell, L., Marti, A., Guzman, J. R., McCreary, M., & Zima, B. (2017). (Re)designing general impression questions to elicit clinically relevant information from children during ADHD medication titration. Oral presentation at *International Pragmatics Conference IPrA*. Belfast, Northern Ireland.

Mikesell, L., Marti, A., Guzman, J. R., McCreary, M., & Zima, B. (2018). Affordances of mHealth technology and the structuring of clinic communication. *Journal of Applied Communication Research, 46*(3), 323–347.

Nova, C., Vegni, E., & Moja, E. A. (2005). The physician-patient-parent communication: A qualitative perspective on the child's contribution. *Patient Education & Counseling, 58*, 327–333.

Oldfield, C., & Fowler, C. (2004). *Mapping children and young people's participation in England.* Research Report RR584. Department for Education and Skills (DfES), Nottingham.

O'Reilly, M. (2006). Should children be seen and not heard? An examination of how children's interruptions are treated in family therapy. *Discourse Studies, 8*(4), 549–566.

Padhilla, S. C. O. S., Virtuoso, S., Tonin, F. S., Borba, H. H. L., & Pontarolo, R. (2018). Efficacy and safety of drugs for attention deficit hyperactivity disorder in children and adolescents: A network meta-analysis. *European Child & Adolescent Psychiatry, 27*, 1335–1345.

Pantell, R. H., Stewart, T. J., Dias, J. K., Wells, P., & Ross, A. W. (1982). Physician communication with children and parents. *Pediatrics, 70*(3), 396–402.

Parry, R. (2009). Practitioners' accounts for treatment actions and recommendations in physiotherapy: When do they occur, how are they structured, what do they do? *Sociology of Health & Illness, 31*(6), 835–853.

Peräkylä, A. (1998). Authority and accountability: The delivery of diagnosis in primary health care. *Social Psychology Quarterly, 61*(4), 301–320.

Ringnér, A., Öster, I., Björk, M., & Graneheim, U. H. (2012). Talking via the child. *Journal of Family Nursing, 19*(1), 29–52.

Robinson, J. D. (2003). An interactional structure of medical activities during acute visits and its implications for patients' participation. *Health Communication, 15*(1), 27–57.

Runseon, I., Enskär, K., Elander, G., & Hermerén, G. (2001). Professionals' perceptions of children's participation in decision making in healthcare. *Journal of Clinical Nursing, 10*(1), 70–80.

Runeson, I. Hallstrom, I., Elander, G., & Hermeren, G. (2002). Children's participation in the decision-making process during hospitalizatoin: An observational study. *Nursing Ethics, 9*(6), 583–598.

Sacks, H. (1992). *Lectures on conversation [1964–72]* (2 vols.). Oxford: Basil.

Sandman, L., & Munthe, C. (2009). Shared decision-making and patient autonomy. *Theoretical Medicine and Bioethics, 30*(4), 289–310.

Schegloff, E. A. (2007). *Sequence organization in interaction: A primer in conversation analysis* (Vol. 1). Cambridge, UK: Cambridge University Press.

Stevanovic, M., & Peräkylä, A. (2012). Deontic authority in interaction: The right to announce, propose, and decide. *Research on Language and Social Interaction, 45*(3), 297–321.

Stivers, T. (2001). Negotiating who presents the problem: Next speaker selection in pediatric encounters. *Journal of Communication, 51*(2), 252–282.

Stivers, T. (2005a). Parent resistance to physicians' treatment recommendations: One resource for initiating a negotiation of the treatment decision. *Health Communication, 18*(1), 41–74.

Stivers, T. (2005b). Non-antibiotic treatment recommendations: Delivery formats and implications for parent resistance. *Social Science and Medicine, 60*(5), 949–964.

Stivers, T. (2006). Treatment decisions: Negotiations between doctors and parents in acute care encounters. In J. Heritage & D. W. Maynard (Eds.), *Communication in medical care* (pp. 279–312). Cambridge: Cambridge University Press.

Stivers, T. (2007). *Prescribing under pressure: Parent-physician conversations about antibiotics*. New York: Oxford University Press.

Stivers, T. (2012). Physician-child interaction: When children answer physicians' questions in routine medical encounters. *Patient Education and Counseling, 87*(1), 3–9.

Stivers, T., & Majid, A. (2007). Questioning children: Interactional evidence of implicit bias in medical interviews. *Social Psychology Quarterly, 70*, 424–441.

Stivers, T., Heritage, J., Barnes, R. K., McCabe, R., Thompson, L., & Toerien, M. (2017). Treatment recommendations as actions. *Health Communication, 33*(11), 1335–1344.

Stivers, T., Sidnell, J., & Bergen, C. (2018). Children's responses to questions in peer interaction: A window into the ontogenesis of interactional competence. *Journal of Pragmatics, 124*, 14–30.

Tannen, D., & Wallat, C. (1986). Medical professionals and parents: A linguistic analysis of communication across contexts. *Language in Society, 15*, 295–312.

Tannen, D., & Wallat, C. (1987). Interactive frames and knowledge schemas in interaction: Examples from a medical examination/interview. *Social Psychology Quarterly, 50*, 205–216.

Tates, K., & Meeuwesen, L. (2000). 'Let mum have her say': Turn taking in doctor-parent-child communication. *Patient Education and Counseling, 40*(2), 151–162.

Tates, K., & Meeuwesen, L. (2001). Doctor-parent-child communication: A (re)view of the literature. *Social Science and Medicine, 52*(6), 839–851.

Tates, K., Meeuwesen, L., Elbers, E., & Bensing, J. (2002). 'I've come for his throat': Roles and identities in doctor-parent-child communication. *Child Care Health Development, 28*(1), 109–116.

ten Have, P. (1991). Talk and institution: A reconsideration of the 'asymmetry' of doctor-patient interaction. In D. Boden & D. H. Zimmerman (Eds.), *Talk and social structure: Studies in ethnomethodology and conversation analysis* (pp. 138–163). Cambridge: Polity Press.

Tiffenberg, J., Wood, E., Alonso, A., Tossuti, M., & Vincente, M. (2000). A randomized trial of ACINDES: A child centered training model for children with chronic illnesses (asthma and epilepsy). *Journal of Urban Health, 77*(2), 280–297.

Toerien, M., Shaw, R., Duncan, R., & Reuber, M. (2011). Offering patients choices: A pilot study of interactions in the seizure clinic. *Epilepsy Behavior, 20*(2), 312–320.

Toerien, M., Shaw, R., & Reuber, M. (2013). Initiating decision-making in neurology consultations: 'Recommending' versus 'option-listing' and the implications for medical authority. *Sociology of Health & Illness, 35*(6), 873–890.

Vis, S. V., Strandbu, A., Holtan, A., & Thomas, N. (2011). Participation and health—A research review of child participation in planning and decision-making. *Child and Family Social Work, 16,* 325–335.

Von Dolmen, A. M. (1998). Children's contribution to pediatric outpatient consultations. *Pediatrics, 102*(3), 563–568.

Wiering, B. M., Noordman, J., Takes, K., Zwaanswijk, M., Elwyn, G., de Bont, E., … Van Dulmen, S. (2016). Sharing decisions during diagnostic consultations: An observational study in pediatric oncology. *Patient Education and Counseling, 99*(1), 61–67.

Wyatt, K. D., List, B., Brinkman, W. B., Lopez, G. P., Asi, N., Erwin, P., … LeBlanc, A. (2015). Shared decision making in pediatrics: A systematic review and meta-analysis. *Academic Pediatrics, 15*(6), 573–583.

4

Clients' Resistance to Therapists' Proposals: Managing Epistemic and Deontic Status in Cognitive Behavioral Therapy Sessions

Katie Ekberg and Amanda LeCouteur

Joint Decision-Making in Cognitive Behavioral Therapy

The theory underlying Cognitive Behavioral Therapy (CBT) places great importance on joint decision-making between therapist and client (Blackburn & Davidson, 1990; Wright, Basco, & Thase, 2006). Unlike other therapies, the therapeutic relationship in CBT is guided by a specific working alliance referred to as "collaborative empiricism" (Wright et al., 2006) that involves therapists and clients working together to gather data that disconfirm core depressive beliefs or thoughts (Beck, Rush, Shaw, & Emery, 1979). Therapists are also encouraged to engage clients in a highly collaborative process in which there is shared responsibility for aspects such as setting

K. Ekberg (✉)
University of Queensland, Brisbane, QLD, Australia
e-mail: k.ekberg@uq.edu.au

A. LeCouteur
University of Adelaide, Adelaide, SA, Australia

C. Lindholm et al. (eds.), *Joint Decision Making in Mental Health*,
The Language of Mental Health, https://doi.org/10.1007/978-3-030-43531-8_4

goals and agendas, giving and receiving feedback, and putting CBT methods into action, both inside and outside the therapy session (Beck et al., 1979; Neenan & Dryden, 2000; Wright et al., 2006). CBT theory thus encourages therapists and clients to work together to question clients' cognitive distortions and unproductive behavioral patterns, with the aim of revealing opportunities for increased rationality, reduced symptoms of depression, and improved personal effectiveness.

One aspect of CBT in which the working alliance of "collaborative empiricism" is considered particularly important is the technique of "Behavioral Activation." According to CBT theory, Behavioral Activation involves engaging clients in a process of change that is designed to stimulate positive thought and hope, or help them solve a problem (Blackburn & Davidson, 1990). Therapists aim to assist clients in choosing one or two actions that make a positive difference to how they feel, and develop a plan to carry out these actions. Therapists are encouraged to engage clients through the use of Socratic questioning, and while they can help guide clients toward actions that might be helpful, whenever possible therapists are expected to allow clients to make the choice (Wright et al., 2006). In particular, CBT theory suggests asking a series of inductive or open questions—in a form that does not provide proposals/suggestions that the client can accept/reject, but which steer the client toward making the proposal for future action themselves. For example, a therapist might ask: "What action could you take in the next couple of days that would begin to make a difference?" A key reason for encouraging clients to make their own choices about behavioral changes within CBT is to avoid client resistance. Resistance to change on the part of clients is considered a major limiting factor to the success of CBT treatment for depression (Leahy, 2001).

Little is currently known, however, about how therapists and clients come to make their decisions about Behavioral Activation tasks within interaction during CBT sessions. This chapter explores how these decisions are made across the sequence of interaction, with a particular focus on who (therapist or client) makes the initial proposal for a behavioral change, and how this proposal for future action is responded to by the recipient.

Joint Decision-Making in Social Interaction: The Negotiation of Epistemic and Deontic Status

For a joint decision to occur in any social interaction, there must be a proposal from one recipient and an approval and commitment to the proposed future action by another participant (Stevanovic, 2012). Each participant thus has some level of involvement in the decision-making process. In order to be involved in decision-making, each person needs to have sufficient knowledge, as well as rights to make decisions (Stevanovic & Peräkylä, 2012). The extent to which a joint decision is made is thus underpinned by each person's epistemic rights (i.e., rights to knowledge) and deontic rights (i.e., rights to determine future action) over the situation (Stevanovic & Peräkylä, 2012). Within CBT sessions, therapists carry the authority of a professional perspective (the epistemics of expertise), however they only have secondary access to knowledge about a client's life and situation (the epistemics of experience) (Heritage, 2013b). Clients will always have ultimate epistemic access to knowledge of how situations have played out in their lives, and they also have the ultimate right to decide on their behavior in the future.

A growing body of conversation-analytic studies has examined the ways in which participants in interaction attend to and manage their rights and responsibilities in relation to knowledge and information in various settings (e.g., Butler, Potter, Danby, Emmison, & Hepburn, 2010; Heritage, 2010, 2012; Heritage & Raymond, 2005; Land & Kitzinger, 2007; Lerner & Kitzinger, 2007; Raymond, 2010; Raymond & Heritage, 2006; Stivers, 2005). Rights and responsibilities concerning what participants know, and have rights to describe, are explicitly oriented to by participants in conversation (Heritage & Raymond, 2005). The majority of work on the management of epistemic status has been conducted in two local environments of interaction: where participants are engaging in assessments (e.g., Clift, 2006; Heritage & Raymond, 2005; Lerner & Kitzinger, 2007; Raymond & Heritage, 2006; Stivers, 2005) and in question–answer sequences (e.g., Heritage, 2010, 2012; Heritage & Raymond, 2010; Raymond, 2010).

Other recent conversation-analytic research has examined how participants in conversation also attend to their deontic rights and obligations (e.g., Kent, 2012; Landmark, Gulbrandsen, & Svennevig, 2015; Lindström & Weatherall, 2015; Stevanovic, 2013; Stevanovic & Peräkylä, 2012, 2014; Zinken & Ogiermann, 2011). Deontic status is concerned with participants' rights to determine future courses of action, that is, to determine "how the world ought to be" (Stevanovic & Peräkylä, 2012). As with epistemic status, people have varying deontic rights in different contexts, and this status is typically managed by parties in particular ways. For example, *announcing* a decision suggests the speaker has higher deontic status than the recipient, whereas *proposing* a decision claims more equal distribution of deontic status. Recipients' responses may accept or resist the previous speakers' claims about deontic status. Establishing a joint decision involves an interplay of the epistemic and deontic status of the participants. In order to have the right to decide on a future course of action, the participants must also have sufficient knowledge of the context that informs that course of action.

Within medical primary care consultations, researchers in conversation analysis have explored how clinicians and patients manage their epistemic and deontic rights to make decisions about treatments. The ways in which clinicians present treatment options have been described in terms of positioning across a deontic gradient. Some forms of treatment presentation set up a steep deontic gradient in that they involve expressions that limit or constrain patients' deontic rights (e.g., providing a *recommendation* for a particular treatment). Other forms set up a shallower deontic gradient in that they mark the decision as the patients' to be made (e.g., listing *options* for possible treatments). As Toerien, Shaw, and Reuber (2013) demonstrate, option-listing, in comparison to recommending, creates a more open space for the type of response that patients can provide, thus allowing for more patient involvement. However, research has also shown that clinicians sometimes deliver options in ways that are biased toward a particular decision, or that exclude potential options (Landmark et al., 2015; Toerien et al., 2013). This body of research on deontic rights in treatment decision-making indicates that even when professionals use communication practices that appear to involve patients in the decision-making process (e.g., recommending a treatment, rather than making a stronger claim), the extent to which patients are involved can vary and is influenced by many interactional factors. Patients have been observed to resist their deontic right to make a decision by claiming their inferior, or lack of, knowledge relative to the clinician (Landmark et al., 2015). However, in other cases patients have been found to assert their deontic rights to make the ultimate decision to accept or reject a treatment proposal (Lindström & Weatherall, 2015). Joint decision-making is thus a complex interactional task that requires ongoing negotiation by the clinician and patient/client across the consultation/session.

Research Questions

This chapter builds on this prior conversation-analytic work on epistemic and deontic rights in interaction by examining how therapists and clients managed decision-making about clients' future courses of action in real-life, video-recorded CBT sessions. In particular, the analysis aimed to explore (1) how therapists initiated discussions regarding the client's future course of action; (2) to what extent clients were given the opportunity to propose ideas for their future action(s); (3) how clients responded to therapists within these decision-making sequences; and (4) how clients and therapists' epistemic and deontic rights over the clients' experience and future actions were managed within the interaction.

Data and Method

The data for this study is a corpus of 20 audio-recorded CBT sessions involving 9 therapists (1 male and 8 female) and 19 clients (1 male and 18 female, all over 18 years old) who were being treated for depression. One client had two of her sessions recorded (these sessions were with two different therapists). The recordings were collected in a free, university-affiliated clinic in Australia that specializes in CBT treatment. Clients at the clinic have weekly appointments, typically for 8–12 weeks. Each recorded session fell in the middle of the client's course of treatment, with therapist and client having established a therapeutic relationship. Sessions involved one client and one therapist in each case, with an average duration of approximately 56 minutes. The total time for all recorded sessions combined was 16 hours, 46 minutes. The study was approved by the University of Adelaide ethics committee. Recordings were transcribed using the Jeffersonian transcription system (Jefferson, 2004), and analyzed using conversation analysis. The analysis is based on a corpus of 34 extended extracts that involved discussion of behavior change, in which therapists proposed a future course of action for the client.

The Accomplishment of Joint Decision-Making in CBT Interactions

Across the corpus of recorded CBT sessions there was evidence of variation in whether it was the therapist or client who made the initial proposal for the client's future course of action. In some instances, therapists invited clients to propose their own idea (see also Chapter 11). In doing so, the therapists claimed a lower epistemic and deontic status relative to the client. More commonly, however, it was the therapist who made a proposal for a future course of action for the client. These proposals set up acceptance/rejection as the relevant response from the client rather than the more open-ended slot where the client could make their own suggestion. In proposing a course of action, the therapists claimed epistemic and deontic status in relation to the decision about what the client should do. The typical response by clients to these proposals for change from therapists was to resist—typically, again, by asserting their deontic right to be more involved in decisions about their own future behaviors.

Therapists Inviting Clients to Make a Proposal for Future Action

In some instances in the corpus, therapists used information-soliciting questions (e.g., Is there anything you could do…) to invite clients to propose a future action. These questions were designed to prompt clients to provide the first suggestion for a possible change they could implement in their lives. For example, the first extract, below, follows an extended troubles-telling by the client concerning her feelings of being overwhelmed. She is dealing with problems involving her daughter; trying to prepare for Christmas; and not getting enough sleep. The extract begins with the therapist's formulation of the client's trouble (lines 1–5). The therapist's information-soliciting question comes at line 12. In each of the extracts, T = therapist, and C = client.

Extract 1a

```
01 T: SOUNDS LIKE (0.2) um when a lot of things come up (.)
02    [u:m] y'know for you: they kind've get priority over
03 C: [Mm ]
04 C: Umhm
05 T: looking after yourself?
06 C: Mm.
07    (0.3)
08 C: Yeah.
09    (.)
10 C: I guess: (0.5) it's: (.) yeah that does.
11    (0.4)
12 T: Is there anything that you could do ta (0.3) h↑elp with
13    that? Do you think? Over the next couple of wee:ks?
14    (2.8)
15 C: >I dunno just< (.) maybe (0.2) wri:ting in my list a
16    bit of time out time.
17 T: ↑Okay.
```

At the beginning of the extract the therapist is offering a gist formulation (Antaki, 2008) of the client's trouble (lines 1–5). The formulation validates the client's prior troubles-telling, while also focusing the discussion on the topic of the client prioritizing other things over herself. The client provides multiple acknowledgments (*mm* line 2, *umhm* line 4, *mm* line 6, and *yeah* line 8) throughout the therapist's turn, and at line 10, looks as if she is about to expand on the formulation in some way (*I guess: (0.5) it's:*), but then redoes her turn to form another confirmation (*yeah that does*). The therapist then asks the client a question (line 12), which invites her to make a proposal for a course of action that would address her trouble (*Is there anything that you could do ta (0.3) h↑elp with that?*). With this information-soliciting question, the therapist claims lesser epistemic and deontic rights than the client in making a decision for future action. She provides an opportunity for the client to draw upon her own knowledge of the situation in order to generate an idea. Thus, she allows the client the right to make the initial proposal and to be actively involved in the decision-making process (see also Chapter 11 of this volume).

A gap ensues in the interaction here (2.8 seconds, line 14), following which the client begins her next turn with *I dunno*. After some brief hesitation, she then moves to provide an option for behavior change (*wri:ting in my list a bit of time out time*), thus orienting to the preference for provision of information that was set up by the therapist's interrogative. The therapist responds with an *okay* (line 17) that accepts the client's suggestion. In providing this acceptance, the therapist reasserts her involvement in the decision-making process. Not only has the therapist provided the client with an opportunity to suggest a behavior change, but the therapist can then accept the change and thus "have the last word" in the third position. This third-position turn shows the therapist managing her deontic right to accept/reject the client's proposal for future action, thus also maintaining her involvement in the decision-making process.

As the sequence progresses, the decision-making process becomes a more complex, and therapist-guided, interactional accomplishment. The extract below is an extension of Extract 1a.

Extract 1b

```
01 T: An' what particular f↑un activity could you look
02    forward to?
03    (0.6)
04 C: OH maybe jus' watching a d-v-d maybe or jus' goin' out
05    the ba:ck ['n]
06 T:           [O ]kay.
07    (0.6)
08 C: No coz if I go out the back I look at the weeds.
09 T: Heh heh heh
10    (0.2)
11 C: Yeah maybe jus' spend some time with Holly=or even just
12    (0.2)
13 T: go to the beach.=
14 C: =YEAH go down the beach [I reckon.] [Might even d]o
15 T:                         [Yeah     ] [Yea::h.     ]
16 C: that.
```

Here, the client's answer to the therapist's information-soliciting question, which occurs over lines 3–4, is highly qualified. The client produces three suggestions including *maybe jus' watching a d-v-d maybe, jus' goin' out the ba:ck*, or *maybe jus' spending some* time with Holly, her dog. All of these suggestions display a rather weak commitment to engage in an activity. The therapist responds to the client's response with some additional work of negotiation. Instead of waiting for the client to finish her turn at line 11, the therapist comes into complete the client's turn at a point where it is projectable that the remaining component of the turn will be a suggestion of an activity. The client's intra-turn pause provides the therapist this opportunity to enter. Rather than beginning a new turn, the therapist produces a continuation of the client's current turn-construction-unit (TCU) (Sacks, Schegloff, & Jefferson, 1974). Lerner (2004) has demonstrated how such "anticipatory completions" work to achieve a heightened sense of affiliation between participants in interaction, and this is what appears to happen here. Therapist and client are not just sharing ideas; they are sharing turns. Although the therapist has suggested the idea of going to the beach, this has occurred as a completion of the client's turn. Additionally, going to the beach is something that the client had said she enjoys doing 10 minutes earlier in the session. The therapist thus draws on her knowledge of the client (based on the client's telling earlier in the session) to make a proposal for the client's future action. The therapist's deontic right to make this proposal is thus based on her shared knowledge that the client would enjoy going to the beach.

The client responds to the therapist's candidate completion with a loud confirmation, *YEAH*. She then partially repeats the completion, reinstating her epistemic authority over the turn's talk (Lerner, 2004; Stivers, 2005). The client then adds that she *might even do that*. The use of *even* in this formulation highlights that the therapist's completion had not been exactly what the client had intended but that it is accepted anyway. In using an anticipatory completion, the therapist has also been able to achieve affiliation with the client. Rather than making an independent suggestion, it is as though the therapist has "read the client's mind." And the client is able to produce a third-position acceptance of the idea, to reinstate her contribution to the suggested course of action.

In sum, across this sequence, it can be seen that both therapist and client join in the decision-making process. Even when the sequence becomes more therapist-guided (than at the outset with the initial open-ended information-soliciting question), the therapist's proposal for the client to go to the beach is generated from prior knowledge of the client's preferences. The client and therapist remain affiliated across the sequence and there are no signs of client resistance to the therapist's actions. In fact, it would be difficult for the client to show resistance to the proposed courses of action given that she either proposed the activities herself or mentioned the activity as something she enjoyed only 10 minutes earlier in the interaction.

Therapists' Proposals for Future Action and Clients' Resistance

The above sequence can be compared with other, more common, sequences in the corpus where it was the therapist who initially proposed a course of future action without first inviting the client to propose an idea (as seen in Extract 1). Therapists' proposals in this CBT corpus were typically followed by localized, active client resistance. Clients drew on knowledge from previous experience, and of the current troubling situation, to produce reasons for their resistance, thus displaying their primary epistemic access to the situation under discussion. By indexing their superior epistemic authority, clients invoked their deontic right to reject the therapist's proposed course of action.

Extract 2 provides an example. Preceding this extract, the focus of talk for most of the session had been around the problematic behavior of the client's youngest daughter, Leah. The client had claimed that her daughter's behaviour was contributing to her own depression. Following this sequence of troubles-telling from the client, in the extract below, the therapist launches straight into a proposal for future action for the client: that the client have some one-on-one time with Leah, and ask her partner, Pete, to keep her elder daughter, Alison, occupied so that this can happen.

Extract 2

```
T: Do you think you could talk with Pete about (0.4)
   the fact that you are quite worried about Leah and
   y'think it's really importan' for her to have some one
   on one time with you.
   (0.4)
T: and would he mind twice a week (0.6) just (0.7) you
   know (0.5) keeping an ear out in the house.
   (0.2)
C: Yep
T: So that Alison is gonna be, (0.8)
C: Yep see if ye- m (0.6) makes me w↑orried what am I
   going to say to Alison.
   (0.2)
C: you know cos she always feels:: (1.3) that (0.3) n-
   the- she's always seen Leah (2.2) with the over
   extended (0.5) whatever's to get the attention.
   =[So sh]e's always gone (1.1)
T:  [Mmhm ]
T: Yep.
   (0.3)
C: sa- sat back an' ya know every time I've spoken to her
   about it y'know .hhhh (0.8) >like I've< made her aware
   (0.3) m I can see tha' ya sittin back becuz your sister
   needs a little more attention [and ] stuff like that.
T:                               [Mmhm]
C: and that's: y'know jea:::h you know (0.5) doesn' matta
   (0.2) [kind of] thing.=It's okay.
T:       [Mmhm   ]
   (.)
C: [I un]derstand.
T: [Mmhm]
   (0.7)
C: So it would be nice for her tuh (1.2) I ALways seem to
   leave her ou:t becuz: (0.2) the youngest one is: (0.4)
T: Okay.
   (0.6)
C: Yuh know.
```

The therapist's proposal (lines 1–10), framed as an interrogative, is downgraded with an epistemic marker (*do you think*), the use of a low-modal operator (*could*), and downgrading devices (*quite, just*). In designing the proposal this way, the therapist highlights its contingent nature (Curl & Drew, 2008), inviting the client either to accept or reject it in response. In making her suggestion in this way, she thus somewhat shares the deontic right to make the decision with the client

(Stevanovic & Peräkylä, 2012). However, the therapist is the one who provides the initial proposal for future action here, rather than asking the client for her own ideas (as seen in Extract 1) and so, in this way, the therapist displays a higher epistemic and deontic stance in relation to the client's future actions. Deciding to agree with a proposal for future action is not the same as choosing your own action (Pilnick, 2008).

The client's response (across lines 11–37) suggests that she may not be satisfied with the therapists' claimed deontic status, as she seeks to establish a stronger deontic position within the interaction. Her response draws upon specific knowledge about her daughters to resist the preconditions of the proposal. The client's reason for resistance is framed as an inability to comply account (Heritage, 1984): She is unable to accept the proposal because she knows, from experience, that her other daughter (Alison) does not respond well to being left out (see also Chapter 5). The client draws upon several high-modality adjuncts to show that her account is not based on knowledge of one particular occasion, but on her knowledge of how things consistently are (Halliday, 1985; He, 1993). When describing her daughter's feelings toward her sibling, the client uses the adjunct *always* several times across lines 14–17. Then, in her expansion at line 21, the client uses the adjunct *every* to describe occasions when she has tried to talk to her daughter about her younger sister. Again, at line 33, the client states that she *always* seems to leave her older daughter out. In producing her account as a factual and generalized description of what happens in her household, the client displays her superior direct access to knowledge of what everyday life is like in her house, and of how her daughter generally reacts to conversations such as the one the therapist is proposing. By indexing her superior epistemic authority in the domain of her experience, the client is able to invoke her deontic right to reject the therapist's proposed course of action. It is easier for the client to reject the therapist's proposal here, compared to Extract 1, because, rather than inviting the client to provide initial ideas for proposed future action(s), the therapist has instead proposed her own idea. In doing so, she displayed a higher epistemic and deontic stance in an environment where it is the client who has the ultimate epistemic and deontic authority over her own experience and future actions.

Another example can be seen in Extract 3. Prior to this extract, there has been a troubles-telling from the client about her visit to a financial planner who is investigating whether she can buy her own home and thus move out of her parents' house as she is currently experiencing some conflict with her parents. The client has told the therapist that the financial planner will not be reporting back to her until closer to Christmas, which is six weeks away. The fragment follows on from the therapist having delivered a gist formulation (Antaki, 2008) of the client's trouble, which the client has confirmed.

Extract 3

```
T: [Alright] so: (1.7) .hh g↑iven that he: hhh can't let
   you know until Christmas (0.6) an' then even if it's a
   yes: (0.2) there'll still be a kinda bit've a ga:p
   (0.2) [bet]ween (0.2) now and when you could possibly
C:       [Yes]
T: buy a courtyard home [an' get] into it.
C:                      [Yes.   ]
C: Yes.
   (0.2)
T: Is it worth exploring some other al- accommodation
   options?
   (0.4)
C: [Uh:]
T: [so ] that you're not liv↑ing at home?
   (0.4)
C: We:ll not really becuz (0.7) in the six weeks I'm off I
   don't get pai:d.
   (0.2)
T: Oka:y.
```

The therapist first delivers an account for her proposal based upon the client's preceding troubles-telling. Pre-proposal accounts set up the delivery of a subsequent proposal by first stating the problem to be solved (Houtkoop-Steenstra, 1990; Waring, 2007). The therapist's pre-proposal account orients to the delicate nature of delivering the subsequent proposal. The therapist gets acceptance from the client of the candidate stated problem, which provides her with a go-ahead to deliver her proposal. Although the interrogative is grammatically structured for a "yes" response, in launching it with the phrase *is it worth* (line 10), the therapist downgrades her epistemic authority over the issue, relative to the client. However, the therapist is the one proposing the idea here for the client to accept/reject. This sets up a different sequential response to instances in which the client is invited to propose her own ideas for a future course of action.

The therapist completes her incremental turn at line 14, and there is a gap of 0.4 seconds where the client does not respond. When the client takes her turn she begins with *Well* which may be indicative of either a forthcoming complex response or a dispreferred response to the interrogative proposal (Schegloff & Lerner, 2009). In this instance, the *well* preface appears to be a marker of the upcoming dispreferred response given the silences from the client at lines 12 and 15, and the *Uh* preface of the client's abandoned turn at line 13. The client responds to the interrogative with a softened "no" response: *not really*. The client's subsequent account for not accepting the proposal involves a specific reason from her own life as to why she is unable to accept the proposal: *in the six weeks I'm off I don't get pai:d*. This account draws on an aspect of the client's life that the therapist could not have known, and is something that the client has no control over. With this resistive account, the client thus displays her epistemic authority over her experience. The reason provided for the resistance is also a factor that is essential for the proposal to be acted out: the client cannot find new accommodation outside of her parents' home without money. The client thus uses her epistemic authority over the situation to invoke her deontic right to reject the therapist's proposed future action.

In Extracts 2–3, the therapist proposes a suggested course of action to the client without first inviting the client's own ideas. Although the therapists use several interactional resources to downgrade their epistemic and deontic stance within their proposal turns, they still claim epistemic and deontic authority by being the one to propose the future action. In each case, the clients resist the therapist's proposal by providing an account that displays their authority in the epistemics of experience, and thus their ultimate deontic right to reject the proposed course of action.

Discussion

Joint decision-making can be a complex interactional task for therapists as they face the dilemma of needing actively to guide the trajectory of the therapeutic interaction, as well as offering clients the opportunity to be involved in decision-making by conceiving their own idea(s) for change. Although therapists carry professional authority, clients have expertise in relation to their own life experiences. This distinction has been referred to as the "epistemics of expertise" in coordination with the "epistemics of experience" (Heritage, 2013b; Lindström & Weatherall, 2015). When implementing joint decision-making, therapists could risk losing sight of the therapeutic goals of the session. This chapter has shown, however, that there can be consequences for the interaction when therapists propose courses of future action to clients without inviting clients to propose their own ideas in decision-making about behavior change.

This chapter has shown how therapists sometimes use information-soliciting questions to provide clients with an opportunity to suggest behavior change. Such questions positioned the client as the knowledgeable party in the interaction; as the one who would know how to change her own behavior. They thus set up a shallow deontic gradient, allowing the client rights to suggest a behavior change. This type of turn structure has important resonances with the theory underlying CBT (Wright et al., 2006), where joint decision-making is accomplished by therapists engaging clients through the use of Socratic questioning (Wright et al., 2006). Socratic questioning involves asking a series of inductive or open questions in a form that does not provide answers to which the client can respond, but which requires the client's direct input. Extract 1 provided an example of such questioning. Although the therapist guided the negotiation, the client was first provided the opportunity to suggest ideas for future actions. In this way, both client and therapist proposed suggestions for the client's future action, participating in joint decision-making across the sequence. Therapist and client appeared aligned and affiliated throughout these sequences, with little or no hearable signs of client resistance.

It was, however, more typical for therapists to propose their own suggestions for clients' future course of action without first asking for the client's own ideas. In doing so, therapists set up a relatively steeper deontic gradient for the decision-making process, implying that they had the right to tell clients what they should do. Even when therapists attempted to frame their proposals in a way that somewhat shared deontic rights (by designing their proposal as a question, or including epistemic markers), they still claimed a higher epistemic and deontic status by proposing a future course of action based on their own thoughts/ideas, rather than the clients'. In this way, the therapists' proposals set up a more unilateral decision-making process, rather than joint decision-making (Collins, Drew, Watt, & Entwistle, 2005). The therapist had not attempted to acquire the client's opinions or preferences before proposing a suggested course of action. These proposals were typically resisted by clients in ways that asserted their epistemic and deontic authority over the situation. Clients made it clear that they were the ones who had the ultimate right to decide what behavior changes they would implement. As Stevanovic and Peräkylä (2012) have previously shown, second speakers may not be satisfied with deontic symmetry; they often seek to establish a stronger deontic position within interaction. These findings support Pilnick's (2008) idea that, for clients in institutional settings, deciding to agree with a proposal for action is not recognized as the same, and not responded to in the same way, as choosing their own action.

Clients drew on knowledge from previous experience, and of the current troubling situation, to produce reasons for their resistance, thus displaying their primary epistemic access to the situation under discussion. In looking at the detail of clients' resistive accounts, we also identified several resources that were repeatedly used to display this epistemic stance. These resources included high-modality terms and generalized clauses (e.g., I'm sure, always, every) (Halliday, 1985; He, 1993), and direct reported speech (Clift, 2006). In examining clients' resistance to therapists' proposals, we can see the interplay between claims of epistemic and deontic stance. Clients' resistive accounts were grounded in their superior knowledge of their own experience, and this knowledge allowed them to invoke their deontic right to reject specific future actions. In this environment, clients' epistemics of experience could trump therapists' epistemics of expertise. These findings build on developing work on the interplay between deontics and epistemics in interaction (e.g., Antaki, 2012; Heritage, 2013a; Landmark et al., 2015; Lindström & Weatherall, 2015) by illustrating some ways in which epistemic and deontic stance can be managed by parties in second-position resistance responses.

Demonstrated patterns in clients' resistance of therapists' proposals for behavior change have important implications for CBT practice. Analysis has demonstrated that when clients resist, they are not only concerned with rejecting the specific proposed change but also with claiming their epistemic and deontic stance in relation to the matter. Such resistance can obstruct the progression of therapy goals, minimize the degree of success in implementing behavior change, and create a poor relationship between therapist and client (Beutler, Moleiro, & Talebi, 2002; Muntigl, 2013; Safran & Muran, 1996). Therapists might therefore benefit from understanding the subtle implications carried by proposals for behavior change, as clients appear to be sensitive to such issues in the way that they frame their responsive turns.

There are similarities, here, to other healthcare settings such as doctor–patient interactions. Although patients in healthcare settings may be willing to defer to a doctor's specialized medical authority (e.g., see Landmark et al., 2015; Toerien et al., 2013), patients may also sometimes draw upon their deontic authority to resist treatment recommendations, for reasons grounded in the lifeworld of the patient (Lindström & Weatherall, 2015). The findings in this chapter similarly show how the therapy session is a complex epistemic and deontic environment where both parties must manage their own knowledge and rights in relation to the activities being accomplished. Close analysis of the present corpus has shown how the different interactional ways in which therapists structure the client's involvement in the decision-making process for future behavioral change can have significant consequences for the trajectory of the therapy session.

References

Antaki, C. (2008). Formulations in psychotherapy. In A. Peräkylä, C. Antaki, S. Vehviläinen, & I. Leudar (Eds.), *Conversation analysis of psychotherapy* (pp. 26–42). Cambridge: Cambridge University Press.

Antaki, C. (2012). Affiliative and disaffiliative candidate understandings. *Discourse Studies, 14*(5), 531–547.

Beck, A. T., Rush, J., Shaw, B., & Emery, G. (1979). *Cognitve therapy of depression*. New York: The Guilford Press.

Beutler, L. E., Moleiro, C., & Talebi, H. (2002). Resistance in psychotherapy: What conclusions are supported by research? *Journal of Clinical Psychology, 58*(2), 207–217.

Blackburn, I.-M., & Davidson, K. (1990). *Cognitive therapy for depression and anxiety: A practitioner's guide*. Oxford: Blackwell Scientific Publications.

Butler, C., Potter, J., Danby, S., Emmison, M., & Hepburn, A. (2010). Advice implicative interrogatives: Building 'client centred' support in a children's helpline. *Social Psychology Quarterly, 73*(3), 265–287.

Clift, R. (2006). Indexing stance: Reported speech as an interactional evidential. *Journal of Sociolinguistics, 10*(5), 569–595.

Collins, S., Drew, P., Watt, I., & Entwistle, V. (2005). 'Unilateral' and 'bilateral' practitioner approaches in decision-making about treatment. *Social Science and Medicine, 61*(12), 2611–2627.

Curl, T., & Drew, P. (2008). Contingency and action: A comparison of two forms of requesting. *Research on Language and Social Interaction, 41*(2), 129–153.

Halliday, M. A. K. (1985). *An introduction to functional grammar*. London: Edward Arnold.

He, A. (1993). Exploring modality in institutional interactions: Cases from academic counselling encounters. *Text: Transactions of the Society for Textual Scholarship, 13*(2), 503–528.

Heritage, J. (1984). *Garfinkel and ethnomethodology*. Cambridge: Polity Press.

Heritage, J. (2010). Questioning in medicine. In A. F. Freed & S. Ehrlich (Eds.), *"Why do you ask?": The function of questions in institutional discourse* (pp. 42–68). New York: Oxford University Press.

Heritage, J. (2012). The epistemic engine: Sequence organization and territories of knowledge. *Research on Language and Social Interaction, 45*(1), 30–52.

Heritage, J. (2013a). Action formation and its epistemic (and other) backgrounds. *Discourse Studies, 15*(5), 551–578.

Heritage, J. (2013b). Epistemics in conversation. In J. Sidnell & T. Stivers (Eds.), *The handbook of conversation analysis* (pp. 370–394). Sussex, UK: Wiley-Blackwell.

Heritage, J., & Raymond, G. (2005). The terms of agreement: Indexing epistemic authority and subordination in talk-in-interaction. *Social Psychology Quarterly, 68*(1), 15–38.

Heritage, J., & Raymond, G. (2010). Navigating epistemic landscapes: Acquiescence, agency and resistance in responses to polar questions. In J.-P. de Ruiter (Ed.), *Questions* (pp. 179–192). Cambridge: Cambridge University Press.

Houtkoop-Steenstra, H. (1990). Accounting for proposals. *Journal of Pragmatics, 14*(1), 111–124.

Jefferson, G. (2004). Glossary of transcript symbols with an introduction. In G. Lerner (Ed.), *Conversation analysis: Studies from the first generation* (pp. 13–23). Philadelphia: Benjamins.

Kent, A. (2012). Compliance, resistance and incipient compliance when responding to directives. *Discourse Studies, 14*(6), 711–730.

Land, V., & Kitzinger, C. (2007). Some uses of third-person reference forms in speaker self-reference. *Discourse Studies, 9*(4), 493–525.

Landmark, A. M. D., Gulbrandsen, P., & Svennevig, J. (2015). Whose decision? Negotiating epistemic and deontic rights in medical treatment decisions. *Journal of Pragmatics, 78,* 54–69.

Leahy, R. (2001). *Overcoming resistance in cognitive therapy.* New York: The Guilford Press.

Lerner, G. (2004). Collaborative turn sequences. In G. H. Lerner (Ed.), *Conversation analysis: Studies from the first generation* (pp. 225–256). Amsterdam: Benjamins.

Lerner, G., & Kitzinger, C. (2007). Extraction and aggregation in the repair of individual and collective self-reference. *Discourse Studies, 9*(4), 526–557.

Lindström, A., & Weatherall, A. (2015). Orientations to epistemics and deontics in treatment discussions. *Journal of Pragmatics, 78,* 39–53.

Muntigl, P. (2013). Resistance in couples counselling: Sequences of talk that disrupt progressivity and promote disaffiliation. *Journal of Pragmatics, 49*(1), 18–37.

Neenan, M., & Dryden, W. (2000). *Essential cognitive therapy.* London: Whurr Publishers Ltd.

Pilnick, A. (2008). "It's something for you both to think about": Choice and decision making in nuchal translucency screening for Down's syndrome. *Sociology of Health & Illness, 30*(4), 511–530.

Raymond, G. (2010). Grammar and social relations: Alternative forms of yes/no-type initiating actions in health visitor interactions. In A. Freed & S. Ehrlich (Eds.), *"Why do you ask": The function of questions in institutional discourse* (pp. 87–107). New York: Oxford University Press.

Raymond, G., & Heritage, J. (2006). The epistemics of social relations: Owning grandchildren. *Language in Society, 35*(5), 677–705.

Sacks, H., Schegloff, E., & Jefferson, G. (1974). A simplest systematics for the organization of turn-taking for conversation. *Language, 50*(4), 696–735.

Safran, J. D., & Muran, J. C. (1996). The resolution of ruptures in the therapeutic alliance. *Journal of Consulting and Clinical Psychology, 64*(3), 447–458.

Schegloff, E., & Lerner, G. (2009). Beginning to respond: Well-prefaced responses to wh-questions. *Research on Language & Social Interaction, 42*(2), 91–115.

Stevanovic, M. (2012). Establishing joint decisions in a dyad. *Discourse Studies, 14*(6), 779–803.

Stevanovic, M. (2013). Constructing a proposal as a thought: A way to manage problems in the initiation of joint decision-making in Finnish workplace interaction. *Journal of Pragmatics, 23*(3), 519–544.

Stevanovic, M., & Peräkylä, A. (2012). Deontic authority in interaction: The right to announce, propose, and decide. *Research on Language and Social Interaction, 45*(3), 297–321.

Stevanovic, M., & Peräkylä, A. (2014). Three orders in the organization of human action: On the interface between knowledge, power, and emotion in interaction and social relations. *Language in Society, 43*(2), 185–207.

Stivers, T. (2005). Modified repeats: One method for asserting primary rights from second position. *Research on Language and Social Interaction, 38*(2), 131–158.

Toerien, M., Shaw, R., & Reuber, M. (2013). Initiating decision-making in neurology consultations: 'Recommending' versus 'option-listing' and the implications for medical authority. *Sociology of Health & Illness, 35*(6), 873–890.

Waring, H. Z. (2007). The multi-functionality of accounts in advice-giving. *Journal of Sociolinguistics, 11*(3), 367–391.

Wright, J., Basco, M., & Thase, M. (2006). *Learning cognitive-behavioural therapy*. Washington: American Psychiatric Publishing Inc.

Zinken, J., & Ogiermann, E. (2011). How to propose an action as objectively necessary: The case of Polish *trzeba x* ("one needs to x"). *Research on Language and Social Interaction, 44*(3), 263–287.

5

Clients' Practices for Resisting Treatment Recommendations in Japanese Outpatient Psychiatry

Shuya Kushida and Yuriko Yamakawa

Professional Authority and Client Participation

Clients' participation in medical decision-making has been increasingly advocated in the field of psychiatry. It has been argued that client participation can enhance adherence to medication, strengthen the therapeutic alliance, and empower clients in their recovery process (Deegan & Drake, 2006; Hamann, Leucht, & Kissling, 2003). However, the model of shared decision-making (SDM) has not been widely actualized in psychiatric encounters (Goss et al., 2008; Matthias, Salyers, Rollins, & Frankel, 2012). While some

S. Kushida (✉)
Osaka Kyoiku University, Kashiwara, Japan
e-mail: kushida@cc-osaka-kyoiku.ac.jp

Y. Yamakawa
Ibaraki Prefectural University of Health Sciences, Ami, Japan
e-mail: yamakaway@ipu.ac.jp

C. Lindholm et al. (eds.), *Joint Decision Making in Mental Health*,
The Language of Mental Health, https://doi.org/10.1007/978-3-030-43531-8_5

studies have reported clients' desire for greater involvement in decision-making (Adams, Drake, & Wolford, 2007), others have reported clients' willingness to leave the final decision to psychiatrists (De las Cuevas & Peñate, 2014; Eliacin, Salyers, Kukla, & Matthias, 2014).

Past research on medical decision-making has proposed clients' orientation to professional authority and the role of a "good" client as a possible account for their reluctance to actively participate in medical decision-making: clients have a fear of being regarded as "difficult" and of the possible resulting negative repercussions on the future doctor–client relationship (Eliacin et al., 2014; Frosch, May, Rendle, Tietbohl, & Elwyn, 2012; Joseph-Williams, Edwards, & Elwyn, 2014). Clients are reported to cope with this fear by complying with their doctor while searching for information elsewhere to decide whether to take the prescribed medicine, or by turning to someone else for assistance in decision-making (Frosch et al., 2012). Though such strategies may be practically helpful, they underscore the difficulty for clients to exert agency in medical decision-making. At present, however, we know relatively little about how clients' behaviors reflect their orientation to professional authority or about whether this orientation is incompatible with their exerting agency in actual psychiatric decision-making.

This study is an attempt to fill this gap by describing some recurrent practices clients use to resist psychiatrists' recommendations about medication changes in Japanese psychiatry. It will show that while clients consistently avoid intruding into psychiatrists' professional authority, they simultaneously use practices with which they navigate the decision-making sequence toward a decision that is sensitive to their preference and concerns. By examining the contingent process of actual decision-making, we argue that clients' orientation to professional authority does not necessarily eliminate their exerting agency in decision-making. Clients' resistance can be regarded as an important opportunity for enhancing client participation in decision-making.

Conversation Analytic Research on Treatment Decision-Making

In conversation analysis, a large body of research has been conducted about medical decision-making in diverse settings (see Chapter 1). In this body of research, studies on clients' resistance to treatment recommendations have described two kinds of resistance: passive resistance and active resistance (Costello & Roberts, 2001; Koenig, 2011; Stivers, 2005, 2007). Passive resistance is implemented by withholding acceptance using such resources as silence and unmarked acknowledgment. Active resistance is defined as "an action that questions or challenges the physician's treatment recommendation, including proposals of alternative treatments" (Stivers, 2005, p. 52). Unlike passive resistance, active resistance makes the psychiatrist's response relevant. Clients shift from passive to active resistance if doctors do not modify their recommendation in response to passive resistance. In addition to these studies on treatment recommendation, Barton et al. (2016) have described clients' presenting "candidate obstacles" (for example, a lack of time to do regular exercise due to work hours) as a practice for resisting lifestyle advice. Overall, these studies have shown that clients do not always simply comply with doctors' recommendations but may exert agency in the process through which the recommendations and advice emerge as acceptable to them.

Compared to the large body of research on somatic consultations, there has been a small but growing number of conversation analytic studies on psychiatric decision-making. These studies have described the organization of the treatment recommendation phase (Bolden & Angell, 2017), psychiatrists' practices for leading up to and recommending treatment (Angell & Bolden, 2015, 2016; Kushida & Yamakawa, 2015, 2018; Quirk, Chapin, Lelliott, & Seale, 2012; Thompson & McCabe, 2018), and clients' practices for soliciting medication change (Bolden, Angell, & Hepburn, 2019) and requesting treatments (Kushida, Hiramoto, & Yamakawa, 2016). However, no study thus far has focused on clients' resistance to treatment recommendations.

Research Questions

It remains to be investigated whether, like other medical clients, psychiatric clients also exert agency in their responses to psychiatrists' treatment recommendations. The present chapter addresses this task by describing the practices clients use to resist psychiatrists' recommendations of medication adjustments. The research questions are:

1. How do clients resist psychiatrists' treatment recommendations?
2. How do their practices for resistance shape the subsequent decision-making process?

Data and Method

The data for this study were 149 video recordings of return visits, each between 1 and 33 minutes long, to an outpatient department of a private psychiatric hospital in Japan. Nine psychiatrists and 145 clients were involved. Most of the clients have had an ongoing relationship with their psychiatrists for months or years. They have been diagnosed with schizophrenia, major depressive disorder, bipolar disorder, minor mood disorders, neurotic disorders, and other mental disorders. The research was approved by the ethical committee of the hospital. Informed written consent was obtained from all participants. From this data set, we excluded 100 consultations in which the psychiatrist and the client agreed to continue with the current medication because the client's condition was stable (75 cases), when the client initiated a treatment discussion by requesting a treatment (23 cases), or when no medication was prescribed (2 cases). In the remaining 49 consultations, the psychiatrist initiated a treatment discussion by either recommending a medication adjustment or by recommending no adjustment even though the client had reported some problem. In these 49 consultations, we examined all the turns in which the psychiatrist recommended treatment as well as the clients' responses to them.

We identified 17 consultations in which the client resisted the psychiatrist's recommendation in some way.

The video-recorded consultations were transcribed following conversation analytic transcription conventions. In each extract, a word-by-word gloss has been provided only when it is essential for the analysis because of limited space. A list of glossing abbreviations is provided in the Appendix.

Clients' Practices for Resisting Treatment Recommendations

Passive Resistance: Withholding Acceptance

Previous studies on somatic consultations have shown that clients initiate negotiation over treatment by withholding acceptance after the doctor recommends a treatment (Costello & Roberts, 2001; Koenig, 2011; Stivers, 2005, 2007). This type of resistance is passive in that it does not explicitly express resistance or convey grounds for resistance. In our data of outpatient psychiatric consultations, clients also withheld acceptance using resources such as a gap of silence or an unmarked acknowledgment.

Extract 1 is an example of passive resistance through both a gap of silence and an unmarked acknowledgment. The client, who has been diagnosed with dysthymia, is currently being treated with extensive medication. In this consultation, he has complained about having trouble staying asleep. His condition is otherwise basically stable. In Extract 1, the psychiatrist explains the medicinal effect of the sleeping pill called Halcion (lines 01–03) and then recommends a switch to another medicine while looking at the client's chart ("So, a switch to another one that has a longer-lasting effect is what I can do for you.", lines 05–07). This recommendation is formatted as an "offer" (Stivers et al., 2017) using the expression *deki* ("can do", line 07).

Extract 1

```
01 P: harushion tte yappari .hh
      Halcion is, after all,

02    sugu::(0.2) kiite kureru::(.)shi:
      a fast-acting medicine and

03    sugu:(.)me ga same chau kusuri na n desu yo.
      it stops working quickly.

04 C: °hn hn°
       Uh huh.

05 P: .hhh hunde
           and
           And so,

06    sore o  chotto nagame  no mono  ni kaeru
      that OP a.bit  longish LK thing P  switch
      a switch to another one that has a longer-lasting
      effect,

07    tte yuu .hhh koto   wa deki   masu kedo ne.
      QP  say      matter TP can.do AUX  CP   FP
      is what I can do for you.

08    (0.2)(0.3)(0.4)
           ↑___↑
           ((P turns to C.))

09 C: °°a:a°°
      Hmm.

10    (0.8)

11 P: nn yame to(0.2)ki masu?
      Well, you don't want that?
```

Soon after her recommendation, the psychiatrist turns to the client (line 08) and continues to monitor him until the end of line 10. The client remains silent for 0.9 seconds (line 08), produces an unmarked acknowledgment token in a very low voice (line 09), and remains silent for another 0.8 seconds (line 10). The psychiatrist treats these responses as resistant by explicitly asking about the client's unwillingness to switch sleeping pills (line 11). This case illustrates a recurrent pattern in our data, in which the client withholds acceptance of a recommendation, and this is understood as resistance by the psychiatrist.

In addition to silences and unmarked acknowledgment tokens, the anaphoric information receipt *soo desu ka* ("is that so") is also recurrently used to withhold acceptance in our data, as we will later illustrate with Extract 2a. It consists of the anaphoric substitution *soo* ("so"), the copula verb *desu* ("be"), and the question particle *ka.* It is syntactically recognizable as a confirmation request and usually gets a minimal confirmation. However, it does not create strong pressure for a response (Stivers & Rossano, 2010) in that it is pronounced without prominence and with a falling intonation. In terms of its prosody, it is recognizable as a claim of information receipt. Its crucial feature as a resource for resistance lies in the fact that by displaying a mediated access to the content of the prior turn with the anaphoric substitution *soo*, clients treat the recommendation as a piece of information that belongs to the psychiatrist's knowledge domain. By thus addressing only the epistemic aspect of the prior turn, clients postpone taking an explicit stance toward the recommendation. Since this only *postpones* taking a stance, it is possible for clients to subsequently accept the recommendation, and they do so in some cases. As it is placed after a turn that prefers acceptance/compliance, however, it is recurrently treated as resistance-implicative, as in Extract 2a.

Extract 2a is an example of passive resistance using an anaphoric information receipt. The client, who has been diagnosed with schizoaffective disorder, is now being treated with extensive medication including the antipsychotic Zyprexa. In this consultation, he has complained about sweaty palms, depression, and a feeling of his thoughts "leaking." Prior to the fragment, the psychiatrist has solicited recognition of another antipsychotic Abilify, which has previously been prescribed to the client. After receiving the client's recognition, he recommends a switch to it ("Let's start it again.", line 01). Though he keeps looking at the client's chart until he turns to the patient in line 09, he officially creates a moment for the decision (Kushida & Yamakawa, 2015), that is, he makes the client's acceptance or rejection a sequentially relevant next action, using the "let's" form in line 01.

Extract 2a

```
01 P: =.hhh >are< o  chotto mooichido hajime mashoo.
            that  OP a.bit  again      start  let's
            Let's start it ((=Abilify)) again.

02      (1.2)

03 C: soo desu ka.
      so  C    Q
      Is that so.

04 P: nn.
      Yeah.

05      (1.0)

06 P: ne,.hh ano ebirifai no hoo       ga::,(0.8)
      FP      uhm Abilify  LK direction SP
      Y'know, 'cause Abilify has,

07    jipurekisa ni kuraberu to::(.)
      Ziprexa     P  compare  CP
      compared with Zyprexa,

08    ano:: hitotsu wa:(.)↑koo       (1.3)
      uhm    one      TP     like.this
      for one thing,

09    <chinsee kooka> ga sukunai kara.
      sedative effect SP small   'cause
      a less sedative effect.
          ↑_↑
      ((P turns to C.))
```

The client first remains silent for 1.2 seconds (line 02) and then produces an anaphoric information receipt *soo desu ka* ("is that so," line 03). The psychiatrist confirms it (line 04), and thereby provides the client with another opportunity to respond to the recommendation. Seeing that the client remains silent for 1 second (line 05), the psychiatrist starts pursuing acceptance by explaining one reason he recommends switching to Abilify ("Y'know, 'cause Abilify has, compared with Zyprexa, for one thing, a less sedative effect.", lines 06–09). He thereby treats the client's prior conduct as resistant. As this case illustrates, the anaphoric information receipt treats the prior turn only as a piece of information (to be confirmed), and thereby enables the client to postpone taking an explicit stance toward the recommendation.

This section has illustrated that clients initially resist treatment recommendations passively by withholding acceptance. What is common to the resources used to do so is that they do not convey anything about what is problematic about the recommendation or the grounds for resistance. By withholding acceptance, clients leave it to the psychiatrist to figure out why the recommended treatment is problematic and to choose how to proceed with the decision-making. Clients exert agency in that they resist the recommendation, but the agency is minimal in that they do not shape the way in which the psychiatrist responds to their resistance.

Active Resistance: Questioning the Recommendation and Revealing a Reason for the Resistance

Clients in somatic consultations have been shown to shift from passive to active resistance when the recommendation they have passively resisted is not satisfactorily amended despite their passive resistance (Costello & Roberts, 2001; Koenig, 2011; Stivers, 2005, 2007). This is also the case with outpatient psychiatric consultations (see also Thompson & McCabe, 2018). In this section, we describe two practices recurrently used for more active resistance, *questioning the recommendation* and *revealing a reason for the resistance*, to show how clients exert more agency in shaping the trajectory of decision-making.

Questioning the recommendation refers to a turn designed as an inquiry into the effectiveness of a recommended treatment or its alternatives. This practice has two features relevant to the way it shapes the subsequent interaction. First, while it focuses on a matter that falls within the psychiatrist's knowledge domain (for example, the recommended treatment and its possible alternatives), it is always designed as an interrogative and thus displays the client's subordinate epistemic stance toward the matter. Second, by inquiring into an aspect of the recommendation, it narrows down what is problematic about the recommendation. This practice invites the psychiatrist to provide an account of the narrowed aspects of the recommendation and to thereby make it more acceptable.

Extract 2b, which is a continuation of 2a, is one example of questioning the recommendation. As mentioned above, the client resists the proposed switch from Zyprexa to Abilify, and the psychiatrist pursues acceptance by explaining the reason for the recommendation (in lines 06–09 and the omitted 29 lines).

Extract 2b
06 P: ne,.hh ano ebirifai no hoo ga::,(0.8)
Y'know, 'cause Abilify has,

07 jipurekisa ni kuraberu to::(.)
compared with Zyprexa,

08 ano:: hitotsu wa:(.)↑koo (1.3)
for one thing,

09 <chinsee kooka> ga sukunai kara.
a less sedative effect.

((29 lines omitted where the psychiatrist further explains the reason for the recommendation.))

39 P: .hhh >dakara ↑chotto sono:< (0.6) ebirifai: (0.2)
So, ((let's try)) Abilify

40 ni: (.) ano mooichido chotto kaete mi mashoo.
let's try ((it)) again.

41 (0.3)

42 C: **ebirifai tte yuu no o nome ba:,**
Abilify QP say N OP take if
If I take this Abilify,

43 P: nn.
Uh huh.

44 (0.4)

45 C: **ii kanji ni (.) kii[te ki masu ka ne:]**
good feeling P work come AUX Q FP
will it work well?

46 P: [ebirifai wa:]: ano::
Abilify has

47 chinsee kooka ga sukunai kara su:go:ku.
an extremely small sedative effect, y'know.

((6 lines omitted where the psychiatrist explains that Abilify probably has the least sedative effect among antipsychotics.))

```
54 P: ano: huyashi temo:: (0.3) koo gyaku ni:(0.3)
      So even if you take a higher dosage,

55    kibun o otoshi te shimau >to yuu koto ga< nai kara.
      it won't make you feel down.

56 C: a::[a.]
      Oh.
```

After the explanation, the psychiatrist reissues the recommendation ("So, ((let's try)) Abilify" "let's try ((it)) again.", lines 39–40). In response, the client upgrades his resistance by questioning the recommended treatment ("If I take this Abilify, will it work well?", lines 42, 45). He displays an unconvinced stance toward the recommendation in two ways. First, though it is not clear what he is referring to with the phrase "work well", he explicitly asks a question about the effectiveness of the recommended medication. Second, he downplays his familiarity with the drug, which he has previously claimed to recognize (see the description before Extract 2a), by using the "name-quoting descriptor" (Kushida, 2015) in referring to it (*ebirifai tte yuu no*, "this Abilify", line 42).

The psychiatrist starts to re-explain the reason for his recommendation immediately after the client's question becomes recognizable in mid-turn ("Abilify has an extremely small sedative effect, y'know.", lines 46–47). He also upgrades his positive assessment of the effects of Abilify (from "less sedative effect", line 09, to "extremely small sedative effect", line 47). Both in terms of position and composition, he uses stronger resources to pursue acceptance. After elaborating on his re-explanation a little more (the omitted 6 lines), the psychiatrist provides its upshot by linking the effects of Abilify to the client's complaint about depression ("so even if you take a higher dosage, it won't make you feel down.", lines 54–55). Though he repeats the same positive assessment of Abilify, it is paraphrased here in a way that clarifies Abilify's relevance to the client's complaint (cf. "client-attentive account", Angell & Bolden, 2015). On hearing this, the client claims understanding using a change-of-state token (Heritage, 1984) *a::a* ("Oh.", line 56), and subsequently accepts the recommendation (data not shown). As this case illustrates, clients can upgrade resistance by questioning the recommendation when the psychiatrist's recommendation does not emerge as acceptable despite their prior passive resistance. And because this practice narrows down the aspect of the recommendation that is problematic to the client, it invites the psychiatrist to account for the narrowed aspects of the recommendation in pursuit of its acceptance.

Another practice used to resist a recommendation actively is *revealing a reason for the resistance.* This refers to a turn in which the ineffectiveness or possible negative effects of the recommended treatment are formulated as the client's actual or hypothetical experiences. Three points should be noted regarding this practice. First, it conveys what is problematic about the recommendation in an explicit way. Second, by formulating the reason for resistance as the client's own experience, clients avoid intruding into the psychiatrist's professional authority. Third, however, since this practice focuses on what falls within the client's epistemic territory, the psychiatrist needs to incorporate the reason into their understanding of the client's situation. Thus, it invites the psychiatrist to reconsider the recommendation in terms of the manageability of the formulated reason for resistance. To the extent that this is unmanageable by the psychiatrist, it can put the psychiatrist in a dilemma: if they further pursue acceptance of the recommendation, they might risk appearing to be insensitive to the client's concerns.

Extract 3 illustrates this dilemma. The client, who has been diagnosed with panic disorder, is currently being treated with the antidepressant Paxil. In this consultation, he says that he experienced extreme anxiety the night before yesterday and has been so depressed since then that he is wondering how he can control his feelings on a day-to-day basis. Without addressing the client's interest in self-control, the psychiatrist recommends that he take a higher dosage of Paxil. The client resists this passively through a gap of silence and an anaphoric information receipt. The psychiatrist subsequently pursues acceptance for approximately two minutes by interweaving two kinds of explanations: that a higher dosage is desirable in order to control the possible reversions in the recovery process of the client's disease; and that the client needs medication because he cannot control his feelings through willpower in the first place. However, the client continues to resist by inquiring into the effectiveness of continuing the current dosage. In Extract 3, the psychiatrist steps out of her epistemic territory by treating the infeasibility of controlling one's feelings through willpower as a matter that everyone knows ("in fact it is difficult, y'know, to do things like that." "to control your condition through willpower.", lines 01–02 and 04). By thus soliciting the client's agreement with what everyone knows, the psychiatrist upgrades the pressure to accept the recommendation.

Extract 3

```
01 P: sonna:- anmari:- ano:: (1.2) muzukashii yo ne.
      in fact it is difficult, y'know,

02    soo yuu no tte ne.=
      to do things like that.

03 C: =[.hhhh      ]

04 P: =[kimochi no] mochi yoo de toka tte °(yuu no wa)°.
        to control your condition through willpower.

05 C: maah soo:: desu yo [ne:.=tada]:: =
      well so    C    FP  FP   but
      Well, that's true.=But on the other hand,

06 P:                    [nn.      ]
                          Yeah.

07 C: =kusuri   ga agaru tte yuu koto  [de::,    ]
      medicine  SP rise  QP  say matter P
      when I think about taking a higher dosage,

08 P:                                  [°n.  n.°]
                                         Uh huh.

09    (1.3)

10 C: yokee         huan    ni nacchau
      all.the.more anxiety P  become
      that makes me more anxious,

11    tokoro ari   masu ne:.
      part   exist AUX  FP
      I have that kind of tendency.

12 P: hn:::::n.
      Hmmm.
```

((13 lines omitted where the client adds that he is worried about taking 30 milligrams, because it is near the maximum amount.))

```
26 P: doo shi yo kka na↓:: (0.3).hhh (0.4) °n::::° (1.2)
      What should I do? uh:::m

27    ja mo↑o chotto yoosu miru?=
      So shall we continue on the current dosage and
      see how it works?

28    =ototoi no hanashi na node.
      'Cause it was only two days ago that you got
      worse.
```

It is at this point that the client reveals a reason for his resistance. After a proforma agreement ("Well, that's true.", line 05), he describes his anxiety about the idea of taking a higher dosage itself ("But on the other hand, when I think about taking a higher dosage, that makes me more anxious, I have that kind of tendency.", lines 05, 07, 10–11). Since this possible negative effect appears to be beyond the control of the psychiatrist, she faces a dilemma between pursuing acceptance and displaying sensitivity to the client's concern. She displays her orientation to this dilemma by displaying reconsideration of the recommendation ("What should I do? uh:::m,", line 26). And she copes with it by making a concession to the client without completely yielding to the client's preference: first, she modifies her recommendation into a *try* at the continued current dosage to "see how it works" ("So shall we continue on the current dosage and see how it works?", line 27); second, she gives an independent reason ("'Cause it was only two days ago that you got worse.", line 28) for the modified recommendation. This case thus illustrates the fact that the practice of revealing a reason for the resistance can sometimes urge the psychiatrist to modify the recommendation so that it becomes acceptable to the client.

In this section, we have shown that by shifting from passive to active resistance, clients exert more agency in shaping the subsequent decision-making trajectory. While clients' practices for withholding acceptance leave it to the psychiatrist to choose how to proceed with the decision-making, their two practices for active resistance convey what is problematic about the recommendation in one way or another and thereby enable the psychiatrist to proceed with the decision-making in particular ways. Clients thus exert more agency in navigating the treatment discussion toward an acceptable outcome.

Resistance to Premature Recommendations: Describing Additional Concerns

Once clients passively resist the recommendation by withholding acceptance, through their active resistance, they typically continue to treat the recommended treatment as problematic in its current form. In a few cases, however, the client goes on to resist not so much the recommended treatment itself as the process through which it has been issued. In this section, we show that the practice of *describing additional concerns* treats the treatment recommendation as premature. *Describing additional concerns* refers to a turn in which the client describes aspects of their overall problem which have not yet been addressed by the psychiatrist. It treats the recommendation as premature in that it redirects the psychiatrist back toward the problem. It invites the psychiatrist to take into consideration some additional aspects of the client's problem in proceeding with the decision-making.

Extract 4 is an example of describing additional concerns. The client, who has been diagnosed with bipolar disorder, is currently being treated with extensive medication including the mood stabilizer Sodium Valproate. He first says that his condition is a little depressed and stable. The psychiatrist asks a series of questions and finds out that, rather than having been stable, the client has experienced a good deal of fluctuation within a day. Subsequently, he recommends increasing the dosage of Sodium Valproate. The client first resists this passively through a gap of silence. The psychiatrist pursues acceptance by explaining the reason for the recommendation, and re-issues the recommendation ("Why don't we take a higher dosage of Valproate? given your current condition.", lines 01–02).

Extract 4

01 P: Barupuro-san age mase n ka?
Why don't we take a higher dosage of Valproate?

02 ima nojootai de areba.
given your current condition

03 (.)

04 C: **.hhh soo desu yo ne:::.=na[nka]:: (de-) n:::n =**
so C FP FP somehow (but) ITJ
That may be right.=Somehow (bu-) uhm

05 P: [°nn°]
Yeah.

06 C: **=.hhhh (0.4) kazoku ni wa**
family P TP
my family members ((are like))

07 **zuibu::n (0.8) genki na n de nee ke-**
quite good C P C not Q
"you're quite good, aren't you?"

08 nn[:: mitai na](h):(h):(h)=
ITJ like C
((they)) are like.

09 P: [ahhh hah]

10 P: =soo mie chau n ja nai ka na: [to omo tte,]n::n.
You just appear that way in their eyes,
I suppose.

11 C: [n::n.]
Yeah.

12 C: **te:: (0.5) yuu kanji na n desu yo [ne:::.]**
QP say feeling C P C FP FP
or ((that's what)) they see in me.

13 P: [n::n.]
Uh huh.

14 C: **>daka<ra yokee ano: .hhh o:::,**
so all.the more uhm
So, all the more because of that,

15 **asa ni na:nika aru to::,(0.6) n::::n (0.8)**
morning P something exist CP ITJ
when I have something to do in the morning,

16 **nanka koo (.) de↓ki nai to yuu [ka::.]**
somehow like.this can not QP say or
I somehow can't do it, or,
17 P: [°nn] nn°
Uh huh

18 (0.4)

19 C: **yaruki ga: (.) nai- [(.)moo]:::=**
motivation SP not.exist anymore
I have no motivation,

20 P: [°nn nn°]
Uh huh.

21 C: **=okora nai to yuu ka:.**
emerge not QP say or
or I don't even feel like.

22 P: .hh de ippoo de:: sono
And on the other hand,

23 yuugata ikoo no genki na X-san o
your condition is good in the evenings

24 kazoku ga miteru to ↑ne,
and your family memebers know that, so

25 C: n:[:n.
Uh huh.

26 P: [asa deki nai anata o mi te::(0.2)
when they see you who can't do things
in the mornings,

27 C: [(na:n]de de-)=
(Why can't-)

28 P: [mata na-]=namaketeru mita[i na ne::   ]=
they may say that you are being idle,

29 C: [soo soo desu.]=
Exactly.

30 P: =[>soo yuu hanashi ni< na cchau kara::,]
or something like that, so,

31 C: =[so::o nacchau n desu yo ne:]:.
That's what they see.

32 P: n::n.
Yeah.

33 C: na n de::(0.3)ike nai n da tte=
Why can't you go ((to the day care center))?

((45 lines omitted where the client elaborates on his complaint about his family members' lack of understanding of his condition, and the psychiatrist says that it may be difficult even for his wife to understand the client's condition because it is only through a detailed verbal examination that the psychiatrist can assess it.))

79 P: yappari:: (e-)soko wa ne:
After all, y'know,

80 shinsatsu shitsu no naka dakara
it's because you are in the consultation room

81 wakaru bubun tte yuu no mo aru no[de::,
that some aspects of your problem become visible so

82 C: [ha:i hai
Yes, yes,

83 [hai hai.]
Yes, yes.

84 P: [okusan] mo isshoni kite mora ttari suru to ↑ne,
if your wife could come with you,

85 C: n[:n.
Uh huh.

```
86 P:   [ano ii no kamoshirenai kedo
         then she might understand your condition better, but

87      X-san chi oisogashii mitai da kara ne:.
        unfortunately your wife appears to be busy, so.

88      (0.5)

89 C: .thh so:o desu [ne:]:.=
            That's right.
```

The client's response to the re-issued treatment recommendation starts by admitting the reasonableness of the treatment ("That may be right.", line 04). However, he rushes through (Schegloff, 1982) the first possible completion and extends his turn to describe his family member's reaction to his situation ("Somehow (bu-) uhm my family members ((are like)) 'you're quite good, aren't you?' ((they are)) like.", lines 04, 06–08). By transforming his turn into something other than a simple agreement, he starts to actively resist the recommendation.

The psychiatrist initially understands the client's turn as citing a third party's positive evaluation of his condition in order to resist the increased dosage of Sodium Valproate. By trivializing the positive evaluation ("quite good", line 07) as only superficial ("you just appear that way in their eyes", line 10), the psychiatrist defends his recommendation against it. However, it turns out that the client is introducing an as-yet-unaddressed aspect of his problem, which is his family members' lack of understanding of his condition. The client sequentially deletes the psychiatrist's defense by designing his next turn ("or ((that's what)) they see in me.", line 12) as a continuation of the reported speech in line 07. Then, as an upshot of his prior mention of his family members' reaction, he says that his family members' positive evaluation of his condition makes his situation even more difficult ("So, all the more because of that, when I have something to do in the morning, I somehow can't do it, or I have no motivation, or I don't even feel like.", lines 14–16, 19, 21). By describing an aspect of his problem that has not been considered when the psychiatrist first recommends increasing the dosage of Sodium Valproate, the client invites the psychiatrist to reconsider his recommendation so it can emerge as more sensitive to the client's overall problem.

The psychiatrist responds to this in two steps. First, he demonstrates his understanding of the client's overall problem by making an inference about a problematic consequence of the family members' positive evaluation ("And on the other hand, your condition is good in the evenings, and your family members know that, so, when they see you who can't do things in the mornings, they may say that you are being idle or something like that.", lines 22–24, 26, 28, 30). The client treats this as assistance in articulating his complaint on his behalf (Kushida, 2011) ("Exactly. That's what they see.", lines 29, 31), and elaborates on the complaint (line 33 and the omitted lines). Second, the psychiatrist displays his having considered an additional solution: having a consultation in the company of the client's wife ("if your wife could come with you, then she might understand your condition better,", lines 84, 86). However, the psychiatrist immediately invokes the client's wife's busyness as an obstacle and invites the client to consider the feasibility of the additional solution ("but unfortunately your wife appears to be busy, so.", lines 86–87). The client confirms the psychiatrist's understanding of his wife's situation ("That's right.", line 89), and after the fragment, he displays his agreement with the infeasibility of the additional solution by elaborating on his wife's busyness. After that, the psychiatrist re-issues the recommendation, which the client accepts.

In Extract 4, the client uses the practice of describing additional concerns not to disagree with the recommended medication itself but to introduce an as-yet-unaddressed aspect of his problem. In response, the psychiatrist demonstrates his understanding of the client's concern, puts an additional solution on the table, and invites the client to co-examine its feasibility. Through this process, the resulting recommendation emerges as more sensitive to the client's overall problem by now being presented as an outcome of the psychiatrist having considered the client's as-yet-unaddressed concern, although the proposed medication regimen remains the same. This case underscores the fact that clients may resist a treatment recommendation not only because it is problematic, but sometimes because it is prematurely issued before the psychiatrist has properly listened to the client's overall problem.

Discussion

Clients' orientation to psychiatrists' professional authority has been proposed as a possible reason for their reluctance to participate actively in decision-making. To investigate whether and how clients' behaviors in actual decision-making reflect this orientation, this study has examined clients' practices for resisting treatment recommendation in Japanese outpatient psychiatric consultations. It has described practices used by clients to resist a recommendation and has shown how they shape decision-making in different ways: withholding acceptance does not display any grounds for resistance and completely leaves it to the psychiatrist to choose how to proceed with the decision-making; questioning the recommendation narrows down problematic aspects of the recommendation and solicits the psychiatrist's explanation about those aspects; revealing a reason for the resistance explicitly conveys grounds for resistance and invites the psychiatrist to reconsider the recommendation in terms of the manageability of the reason for resistance; and describing additional concerns suggests the prematurity of the recommendation and invites the psychiatrist to take into consideration some additional aspects of the client's problem in proceeding with the decision-making.

What is common to these practices is that clients resist the recommendation without explicitly challenging the psychiatrist's authority. Clients either display their subordinate epistemic stance toward the matter when they focus on something that falls within the psychiatrist's knowledge domain or avoid intruding into the psychiatrist's epistemic territory by formulating possible obstacles for accepting the recommendation as something that falls within their own epistemic territory. Clients thus consistently display respect to psychiatrists' authority even though they resist their recommendations. In a sense, this finding is compatible with the argument put forward in previous studies, that because clients have a fear of being regarded as "difficult," they avoid a gamble that might threaten their future relationship with the psychiatrist (Frosch et al., 2012; Joseph-Williams et al., 2014).

However, this study has also provided evidence that clients' behaviors in actual decision-making are not necessarily characterized by "passivity and compliance" (Joseph-Williams et al., 2014, p. 1). Rather, clients have been shown to exert agency in navigating treatment discussions toward an outcome that reflects their preference and concerns. Clients typically start resisting by withholding acceptance, which is the weakest form of resistance in shaping the subsequent interaction. When an acceptable recommendation does not subsequently emerge, however, the client uses practices such as questioning the recommendation, revealing a reason for the resistance, or describing additional concerns, each of which then shapes the subsequent interaction in a specific way. By ordering their practices for resistance in this way, clients adjust the agency they exert for each sequential environment such that they minimize the risk of being regarded as challenging the psychiatrist's authority, while simultaneously maximizing the chance that the resulting recommendation will become more sensitive to their concerns. In this study, we have demonstrated that the previous findings on clients' resistance in other medical settings (Barton et al., 2016; Costello & Roberts, 2001; Koenig, 2011; Stivers, 2005, 2007) basically hold for routine outpatient psychiatric consultations as well. In addition, it has enhanced our understanding of clients' resistance by describing different ways in which their practices for resistance shape the subsequent trajectory of decision-making. It remains to be investigated, however, whether the finding holds for other types of psychiatric encounters such as those with inpatients or clients in crisis.

The findings have two practical implications. First, clients' resistance can be regarded as an important opportunity to enhance clients' participation (cf. Barton et al., 2016), rather than as a trouble to be eliminated. Our analysis provides evidence that once clients start resisting with the weakest practices, they often continue to resist until their concerns are addressed by the psychiatrist. Therefore, it would be desirable for psychiatrists in time-limited outpatient consultations to ask questions about the client's concerns at the first indication of resistance, so they can start involving the client in the decision-making and adjusting their recommendations to the client's perspective earlier (cf. Koenig, 2011). Second, the analysis of Extract 4 illustrates the fact that clients sometimes resist not so much the content of the recommendation as the *process* in which it is embedded. It would be fruitful to encourage psychiatrists to reflect on not only what they recommend and how they design their recommendations, but also on the process that leads up to the recommendation and their displayed sensitivity therein.

Acknowledgments This study was funded by JSPS KAKENHI Grant Numbers 20200043, 21530496, 23330183, and 24530623.

References

Adams, J. A., Drake, R. E., & Wolford, G. L. (2007). Shared decision-making preferences of people with severe mental illness. *Psychiatric Service, 58*(9), 1219–1221.

Angell, B., & Bolden, G. B. (2015). Justifying medication decisions in mental health care: Physicians' accounts for treatment recommendations. *Social Science and Medicine, 138,* 44–56.

Angell, B., & Bolden, G. B. (2016). Team work in action: Building grounds for psychiatric medication decisions in assertive community treatment. In M. O'Reilly & J. Lester (Eds.), *Handbook of adult mental health: Discourse and conversation studies* (pp. 371–393). London: Palgrave Macmillan.

Barton, J., Dew, K., Dowell, A., Sheridan, N., Kenealy, T., Macdonald, L., … Stubbe, M. (2016). Patient resistance as a resource: Candidate obstacles in diabetes consultations. *Sociology of Health & Illness, 38*(7), 1151–1166.

Bolden, G. B., & Angell, B. (2017). The organization of the treatment recommendation phase in routine psychiatric visits. *Research on Language and Social Interaction, 38*(4), 451–479.

Bolden, G. B., Angell, B., & Hepburn, A. (2019). How clients solicit medication changes in psychiatry. *Sociology of Health & Illness, 41*(2), 411–426.

Costello, B. A., & Roberts, F. (2001). Medical recommendations as joint social practice. *Health Communication, 13*(3), 241–260.

Deegan, P. E., & Drake, R. E. (2006). Shared decision making and medication management in the recovery process. *Psychiatric Services, 57*(11), 1636–1639.

De las Cuevas, C., & Peñate, W. (2014). Preferences for participation in shared decision making of psychiatric outpatients with affective disorders. *Open Journal of Psychiatry, 4*(1), 16–23.

Eliacin, J., Salyers, M. P., Kukla, M., & Matthias, M. S. (2014). Factors influencing patients' preferences and perceived involvement in shared decision making in mental health care. *Journal of Mental Health, 24*(1), 24–28.

Frosch, D. L., May, S. G., Rendle, K. A. S., Tietbohl, C., & Elwyn, G. (2012). Authoritarian physicians and patients' fear of being labeled "difficult" among key obstacles to shared decision making. *Health Affairs, 31*(5), 1030–1038.

Goss, C., Moretti, F., Mazzi, M. A., Piccolo, L. D., Rimondini, M., & Zimmermann, C. (2008). Involving patients in decisions during psychiatric consultations. *The British Journal of Psychiatry, 193*(5), 416–421.

Hamann, J., Leucht, S., & Kissling, W. (2003). Shared decision making in psychiatry. *Acta Psychiatrica Scandinavica, 107*(6), 403–409.

Heritage, J. (1984). A change-of-state token and aspects of its sequential placement. In J. M. Atkinson & J. Heritage (Eds.), *Structures of social action: Studies in conversation analysis* (pp. 299–345). Cambridge: Cambridge University Press.

Joseph-Williams, N., Edwards, A., & Elwyn, G. (2014). Power imbalance prevents shared decision making. *British Medical Journal, 348,* g3178.

Koenig, C. J. (2011). Patient resistance as agency in treatment decisions. *Social Science and Medicine, 72*(7), 1105–1114.

Kushida, S. (2011). Confirming understanding and acknowledging assistance: Managing trouble responsibility in response to understanding check in Japanese talk-in-interaction. *Journal of Pragmatics, 43*(11), 2716–2739.

Kushida, S. (2015). Using names for referring without claiming shared knowledge: Name-quoting descriptors in Japanese. *Research on Language and Social Interaction, 48*(2), 230–251.

Kushida, S., Hiramoto, T., & Yamakawa, Y. (2016). Patients' practices for taking the initiative in decision-making in outpatient psychiatric consultations. *Communication & Medicine, 13*(2), 169–184.

Kushida, S., & Yamakawa, Y. (2015). Fitting proposals to their sequential environment: A comparison of turn designs for proposing treatment in ongoing outpatient psychiatric consultations in Japan. *Sociology of Health & Illness, 37*(4), 522–544.

Kushida, S., & Yamakawa, Y. (2018). Steering interactions away from complaints about persistent symptoms in psychiatric consultations. *East Asian Pragmatics, 3*(1), 91–123.

Matthias, M. S., Salyers, M. P., Rollins, A. L., & Frankel, R. M. (2012). Decision making in recovery-oriented mental health care. *Psychiatric Rehabilitation Journal, 35*(4), 305–314.

Quirk, A., Chapin, R., Lelliott, P., & Seale, C. (2012). How pressure is applied in shared decisions about antipsychotic medication: A conversation analytic study of psychiatric outpatient consultations. *Sociology of Health & Illness, 34*(1), 95–113.

Schegloff, E. A. (1982). Discourse as an interactional achievement: Some uses of "uh huh" and other things that come between sentences. In D. Tannen (Ed.), *Analyzing discourse* (pp. 71–93). Washington, DC: Georgetown University Press.

Stivers, T. (2005). Parent resistance to physicians' treatment recommendations: One resource for initiating a negotiation of treatment recommendation. *Health Communication, 18*(1), 41–74.

Stivers, T. (2007). *Prescribing under pressure: Parent-physician conversations and antibiotics*. New York: Oxford University Press.

Stivers, T., Heritage, J., Barnes, R. K., McCabe, R., Thompson, L., & Toerien, M. (2017). Treatment recommendations as actions. *Health Communication, 33*(11), 1335–1344.

Stivers, T., & Rossano, F. (2010). Mobilizing response. *Research on Language and Social Interaction, 43*(1), 3–31.

Thompson, L., & McCabe, R. (2018). How psychiatrists recommend treatment and its relationship with patient uptake. *Health Communication, 33*(11), 1345–1354.

6

Taking a Proposal Seriously: Orientations to Agenda and Agency in Support Workers' Responses to Client Proposals

Melisa Stevanovic, Camilla Lindholm, Taina Valkeapää, Kaisa Valkia, and Elina Weiste

Joint decision-making is regularly launched by a proposal. Inasmuch as these proposals are made by mental health professionals, the genuine jointness of the decision-making outcome is dependent on the degree to which clients can be encouraged to respond to these proposals in their own terms. Thus, from the perspective of equal participation, those situations in which the clients make proposals may come across as optimal. What will be demonstrated below, however, is the complexity of these sequences. This chapter provides an account of the dilemmas that support workers at the Clubhouse mental health rehabilitation community face when seeking to take client's proposals "seriously."

M. Stevanovic (✉) · T. Valkeapää · K. Valkia
University of Helsinki, Helsinki, Finland
e-mail: melisa.stevanovic@helsinki.fi

C. Lindholm
Tampere University, Tampere, Finland
E. Weiste Finnish Institute of Occupational Health, Helsinki, Finland

C. Lindholm et al. (eds.), *Joint Decision Making in Mental Health*,
The Language of Mental Health, https://doi.org/10.1007/978-3-030-43531-8_6

Agenda, Agency, and Client Encouragement

Joint decision-making as an activity is deeply intertwined with control over the agenda of interaction. Besides suggesting a specific idea, every proposal involves an implicit suggestion about what should be done right now—that is, to engage in a discussion about the idea (Stevanovic, 2013, 2015). In this sense, the mere act of making a proposal entails an attempt to exercise control over the agenda of the ongoing interaction. Indeed, proposals constitute effective attempts to counteract what Lukes (1974) referred to as "non-decisions," which result from all those social pressures that discourage the making of proposals about specific issues and lead to their suppression from becoming "decisionable" in the first place.

Control over the interactional agenda is typically associated with institutionalized positions of power and deontic authority (Stevanovic & Peräkylä, 2012), which characterize news interviews (Greatbatch, 1988) and encounters in the classroom (Mehan, 1979) and court (Atkinson & Drew, 1979). In her classical study on family health-promotion encounters, Kendall (1993) found that "the health visitors set the agenda for the visit, controlled 'turn taking' by asking many questions, gave unsolicited advice and managed closure of a conversation" (p. 105). In organizational meetings, there is often an appointed chairperson exerting control over what will be talked about and when (Angouri & Marra, 2011; Boden, 1994), while in informally organized meetings the interactional agenda may be negotiable from moment to moment (Stevanovic, 2013).

Control over the interactional agenda is inherently bound to agency. According to Enfield (2011), the notion of agency denotes "the type and degree of control and responsibility a person may have with respect to their design of communicative actions and other kinds of signs" (p. 304). Drawing on the deconstruction of *speakerhood* by Goffman (1981), Enfield (2011) has argued that the turn-by-turn unfolding of interaction entails a fundamental asymmetry between initiative and responsive actions. This asymmetry consists of the speaker of the initiative action exercising control over the content of the responsive action. Consequently, first speakers may also be held *accountable* for two aspects of their actions: (1) that they are committed to the content of what is being said and (2) that they are committed to the "appropriateness of saying it here and now" (Enfield, 2011, p. 308). From this perspective, a proposal, as any other "first" utterance in a sequence of utterances, is a risky endeavor. It entails claims of sincerity and relevance, the validity of which will be determined intersubjectively in and through the utterances to come.

In this chapter, we examine how support workers respond to clients' proposals during mental health rehabilitation group meetings at one Finnish Clubhouse community. According to Clubhouse standards, membership in a Clubhouse community entails the right and obligation to participate in consensus-based decision-making about all the matters that affect the life of the community (see Chapter 12). Accordingly, support workers exhibit a strong explicit orientation to encouraging clients to participate in joint decision-making. While this orientation is visible in the support workers' attempts to encourage clients to respond to their proposals (see Chapter 2), the same ideal may also be assumed to inform their ways of responding to the clients' proposals. The support workers may want to take the clients' proposals "seriously," not only for the sake of local interactional needs but also in order to encourage further similar participation through positive reinforcement (e.g., Seligman & Csikszentmihalyi, 2000). However, as we will show in the analysis in this chapter, providing an adequate response to a client's proposal is a complex endeavor—one that is intertwined with dilemmas concerning agenda, on one hand, and agency, on the other.

Treatment of Proposals in Joint Decision-Making Interaction

Responding to a proposal can have quite distinct dynamics depending on whether the proposal has been made in a dyadic vs. group conversation. Therefore, we will first discuss the treatment of proposals in dyads. These considerations will provide a background against which the specific dilemmas of responding to proposals in a group conversation can then be highlighted.

Responding to Proposals During Dyadic Interaction

Joint decision-making in a dyad can sometimes be fast. After one participant has made a proposal, a joint decision emerges when the co-participant accepts the proposal—even if the recipients' accepting responses as such involve multiple facets (Stevanovic, 2012; see Chapter 2). What is essential for a genuinely joint decision to emerge is that it is the recipient bears the main responsibility for transforming the proposal into a decision. If the proposer takes a too dominant role in this respect, the jointness of decision-making outcome is compromised (see Chapter 2).

Orientation to the primary responsibility of the recipient to push the proposal sequence forward toward a joint decision has important advantages. First, it gives the proposal recipient the opportunity to reject the proposal de facto simply by refraining from bringing the sequence toward a decision. Second, the possibility of such implicit rejections allows the proposers to "cancel" their proposals by simply refraining from pursuing them anymore in the face of a lack of recipient responsiveness (Stevanovic, 2012). Third, and most relevantly from the perspective of the present considerations, the opportunity to treat proposals in multiple ways allows for subtle negotiations of the participants' joint decision-making agenda. Not everything can or should be decided together but only those matters that belong to the participants' sphere of joint decision-making (Stevanovic, 2013, 2015). Inasmuch as proposal recipients actively respond to their co-participants' proposals "as proposals," they embrace their content into the participants' joint decision-making sphere. In so doing, they also validate the relevance of the proposal in the here and now.

Responding to Proposals During Group Interaction

There are significant differences between how proposals may be treated in a dyad vs. in a group. Specifically, the existence of multiple proposal recipients in a group creates a challenge to construct the outcome of the proposal as a *joint* decision—one to which all the participants would be committed. Thus, instead of moving the sequence actively toward a decision, which would be expected in a dyad, a participant who first responds to a proposal may contrariwise seek to *slow down* the pace of the unfolding activity. In this way, it can be assured that the decision will not get established before every group member has had the opportunity to contribute to it.

The slowing down of the process by which a proposal is turned into a decision is in tension with providing individual proposal speakers recognition for their interactional contributions. While such recognition may be needed in all decision-making, such a need is likely to be particularly prevalent in a group setting, where the mere act of making a proposal involves a claim of the right to exercise control over the group's interactional agenda. Such claims may then be best validated by the other participants becoming actively and enthusiastically engaged with the content of the proposal. This means that in contexts such as ours, the facilitators of interaction must respond to proposals in positive and approving ways.

From the perspective of group dynamics, however, strongly approving responses to proposals may be problematic in that they may imply a final decision (Stevanovic, 2012). In turn, this may discourage other participants from further participation and exclude them from the decision-making process. The other participants would either need to "second" the first recipient's approval of the proposal, or to seek to slow down the process by making the first recipient's "premature" approval of the proposal a target of explicit meta-level reflection, which would require a lot of interactional skills. Therefore, instead of providing abundant praise, the facilitators of group interaction may seek to find other ways to provide individual proposal speakers with recognition of their interactional contributions.

Research Questions

In this chapter, we consider client-initiated joint decision-making sequences during mental health rehabilitation group meetings at the Clubhouse community. Our analysis is guided by two leading questions:

1. How do the support workers respond to the clients' proposals?
2. To what extent do the support workers' different ways of responding open or close opportunities for the other clients to participate in the ongoing decision-making?

Data and Method

The data used in this study consist of 29 video-recorded 30–60-minute-long meetings of a mental health rehabilitation group in a Finnish Clubhouse community. The meetings took place weekly between September 2016 and August 2017. Each meeting was attended to by 2–10 members and 1–3 support workers trained in social work. The data collection was based on the participants' informed consent. Research ethics approval was obtained from the Southern Finland Clubhouse Association (date of the decision: 19.09.2016) and research permission was given by the board of support workers at the Clubhouses in the relevant area.

The meetings involved the participants discussing the clients' competencies from the perspective of their future employment plans. Simultaneously, the meetings also provided a site for the clients to practice their joint decision-making skills, as a typical meeting involved the participants making choices about the kinds of activities that they would carry out in the group. During such relatively low-stakes decision-making processes, the clients were usually given multiple opportunities to make proposals and respond to those of the support workers or other clients.

Methodologically, the study builds on the line of interactionist sociology introduced by Harold Garfinkel (1967) and Erving Goffman (1959, 1967, 1981) and developed by scholars in the tradition of conversation analysis (Schegloff, 2007). While conversation analysis is used to ask how language and other communicative resources are used to accomplish sequences of initiative and responsive actions, our analysis focuses on one form of such a sequence—the proposal-response sequence initiated by a mental health client. In our data, we identified 180 instances of such sequences, which we then examined on a case-by-case manner in our joint data sessions (see Stevanovic & Weiste, 2017). Below, we account for the reoccurring patterns identified in the entire data collection, demonstrating the range of different support worker orientations in response to clients' proposals. Thereby, we also illuminate two dilemmas involved in the support workers' attempts to take client proposals "seriously."

Agenda and Agency in Support Workers' Responses to Client Proposals

We start our analysis of support workers' responses to client proposals by describing these responses with reference to a dilemma that concerns the management of the participants' interactional *agenda*. Thereafter, we analyze these responses in relation to another dilemma, which deals with the distribution of *agency* between the clients and the support workers.

A Dilemma of Agenda: Balancing Between Individual Recognition and Collective Participation

As pointed out above, when designing their responses to client proposals, support workers need to balance between (1) providing individual clients with recognition for their interactional contributions and (2) encouraging collective participation. To increase understanding of this phenomenon, we analyze one example at each of the two extremes.

Extract 1 represents an instance of a support worker's immediate acceptance of a client proposal. Previously at the meeting, the participants—eight clients and two support workers—have discussed whether it would be possible that, in their following meetings, they would engage in some form of self-evaluation. In lines 1–3, one of the support workers (SW1) points to specific material that could be used as a resource during the evaluation activity.

Extract 1

```
01 SW1: voiko olla sit yks semmonen mitä me
        can it then be one such thing that we

02      voitas hyödyntää tässä arvioinnissa (.)
        could make use of in this evaluation (.)

03      oman toiminnan arvioinnissa?
        in the evaluation of one's own action

04      (1.5)

05 Mio: se vois  liittyä          siihen  parina, (0.7)
        it could be.part.of-INF in.that pair-ESS
        it could be part of that pair (0.7)

06      tekemiseen että toinen kyselee vähän.
        do-INF-ILL CP   other  ask     a.bit
        work so that the partner asks a bit

07 SW1: ↑niin (.) sen    vois  tehä   sillai.
        P         it-GEN could do-INF in.that.way
        ↑yeah (.) it could be done like that.

08 Mio: siinä vahvistettas vähän,
        there we would strengthen a bit

09      (3.0)

10 Eki: eli parityöskentelyä.
        so pair work
```

SW1's suggestion (lines 1–3) is first followed by silence (line 4). Thereafter, Mio makes a proposal on how to use the material introduced by the support worker (lines 5–6). He refers to the idea of "pair work" that has been mentioned earlier at the meeting, now applying it to the realization of the self-evaluation activities. SW1 responds by immediately accepting Mio's proposal (line 7), which is followed by Mio giving a justification for it (line 8). After the ensuing silence (line 9) Eki, who has been acting as secretary for the meeting, states aloud the decision to be written on the meeting minutes (line 10). In this way, the decision is treated as established (cf. Chapter 8), after which the participants start to discuss another topic.

Thus, Mio is certainly given recognition for his proposal by the support worker, who immediately accepts it. Simultaneously, however, the support worker's treatment of Mio's proposal allows it to have only limited influence on the participants' interactional agenda. There is little room for the other participants to express their views on Mio's idea. Therefore, Mio's implicit claim that his turn introduces a relevant topic to discuss in the group is left unconfirmed.

Extract 2 represents a reverse example of support workers' treatment of client proposals. During the previous week, all group members have been able to suggest a name for the group by writing it on a board. Now the participants need to decide between the suggested name alternatives—an activity that is explicitly launched by one of the support workers (SW1) in line 1.

Extract 2

```
01 SW1: mitä  me nä[istä  val-
        which of th[ese do we cho-

02 Pia:             [mä  sanon työvalmennusryhmä
                     SG1 say-1 work.couching.group
                    [I say work couching group

03      (.) vois  olla   ninku semmone, (3.0) vähä
            could be-INF P     sort.of        a.bit
        (.) (it) could be like sort of (3.0) a bit

04      help- helppo ninku ymmärtää ja käsitellä.
              easy   P
              easy erm to understand and deal with

05      (5.0)

((lines 06-16 removed))

17      (2.5)

18 Esa: mitäs niin olikaan.
        what were they

19      (0.7)

20 SW1: siirto ↑seitsemäntoista ryhmä (.) valmennusryhmä
        move seventeen group (.) coaching group

21      (.) rukkisryhmä (.) ja työvalmennusryhmä.
        (.) mitten group (.) and work couching group
```

```
22        (0.4)

23 Pia:   no mä  oon   edelleen sitä   mieltä   et se
          P  SG1 be-1  still    it-PAR mind-PAR CP it
          well I am still of the opinion that that

24        työvalmennusryhmä   ois     ehkä    semmonen,
          work.couching.group be-COND perhaps sort.of
          work couching group would perhaps be the sort of

25        (0.4) selkeesti tosta.
                clear-ADV that-ELA
          (0.4) clearly from there

26        (3.7)

27 Pia:   mitä muiden °mielipiteet on°.
          what are others' °opinions°

28        (0.8)

29 SW2:   kertokaa    vähän (.) ajatuksia.
          tell-IMP-PL a.bit     thought-PL-PAR
          tell us a bit (.) (your) thoughts

30         (0.8)


31 SW2:    mikä tuntuu
           which one feels like

32 Pia:   mikäs Ainosta kuulostaa hyvältä.
           which one feels good for Aino
```

Pia is active in taking a stance toward one of the suggested alternatives. Overlapping with SW1's turn (line 1), Pia makes a proposal for the name *työvalmennusryhmä* "work coaching group" (line 2), justifying her choice in the rest of her turn (lines 3–4). What, however, ensues is a long silence (line 5), followed by SW1 asking the group about the background for one name suggestion (lines 6–16, not shown in the transcript). After the side sequence, Esa launches a return to the decision-making activity by requesting epistemic access to what is now to be decided on (line 18). In response to Esa, SW1 lists the four suggested name alternatives (lines 20–21), after which Pia repeats her original proposal (lines 23–25). Pia's proposal is again met with silence (line 26). This time, however, she reacts to the silence by asking explicitly about the opinions of other participants, first generically (line 27) and then by addressing one participant by name (line 32). Pia's questioning is accompanied by SW2's turns with analogous orientation—a concern for encouraging a higher level of group participation (lines 29 and 31).

Thus, in Extract 2, the support workers, and finally also the proposal speaker, share an orientation to a need of the clients other than Pia to express their opinions about the choice to be made. However, this way of maintaining participation opportunities for the other clients occurred at Pia's cost, because she received no support worker recognition for her proposal.

In a dyad, a proposal recipient can take the decision-making sequence quickly to a close without jeopardizing the jointness of the decision-making outcome (Stevanovic, 2012). However, the situation is different in a group. As demonstrated in the analysis of Extracts 1–2, a sufficiently slow progression of decision-making is a prerequisite for being able to involve several participants in the discussion and thus to establish anything that resembles a joint decision. Therefore, the mere act of making a proposal in a group involves a claim of the right to determine the participants' interactional agenda for *longer* than would most likely be the case in a dyad. A need to offer recognition to proposal speakers for their interactional contributions may thus be even more acute than in a dyad. Paradoxically, however, in a group, the provision of such recognition may go against the dynamics of collective participation.

A Dilemma of Agency: The Paradox of Other- and Self-Orientation in Responses to Proposals

Taking a stance toward a proposal requires that the participants have enough knowledge to understand what it is about. Such epistemic access can be established in different ways, exhibiting different distributions of agency between the proposers and recipients. In responses that may be described as *other-oriented*, the recipient makes the proposer the focus of attention, asking about his or her views, interests, wants, and needs (Svennevig, 2014, p. 316). In contrast, with responses that may be labeled as *self-oriented*, the recipient states his or her own thoughts about the proposal, thus implicitly claiming epistemic access to it. Between these two extremes, there is a continuum of different mixtures of self- and other-orientation. In this section, we will consider the paradoxical consequences that different distributions of agency exhibited in the support workers' responses to client proposals have for the participation dynamics of the group.

Extract 3 represents an instance of *other-orientation*. It is from a meeting at which the participants plan the program for the entire autumn season. In lines 1–3, Ere makes a proposal.

Extract 3

```
01 Ere: pareina     vois  olla   hyvä lähtee hakemaan
        pair-PL-ESS could be-INF good go-INF search-INF-ILL
        it would be to go as pairs to seek

02      työvoimatoimistosta   ninku uutta (-)
        employment.agency-ELA P    new-PAR
        from the employment agency like new (-)

03      (2.0) opetusta     °siitä°,
              teaching-PAR about.it
        (2.0) teaching °about it°

04      (1.5)

05 SW1: tarkotiksä     et vois  tuoda     tähän   ryhmään
        mean-PST-2+SG2 CP could bring-INF to.this group-ILL
        did you mean that one could bring to this group

06      siis jotain, (1.0) tiettyjä       aiheita
        P    something     specific-PL-PAR topic-PL-PAR
        like some, (1.0) specific topics

07      sieltä,
        from.there
        from there

08 Ere: pareina     tai ryhmässä (1.5) vois hakee (.)
        pair-PL-ESS or  group-INE        could search-INF
        as pairs or in a group (1.5) (we) could search (.)

09      nettisivuilta, (1.4) minkälaista (-) esimerkiks
        website-PL-ABL       what.kind.of    for.example
        from websites, (1.4) how for example

10      on työt    jossain   muual ku,
        be work-PL somewhere else  P
        work is like somewhere else than
```

```
11        (3.0)

12 SW2:  kuulenks mä  Ereä     oikein et sä  toivoisit
         hear-1-Q SG1 Name-PAR right CP SG2 wish-COND-2
         do I hear Ere correctly that you would wish for

13       sellasta    tietoa          et mitä se työ (.)
         sort-of-PAR information-PAR CP what it work
         the sort of information about what the work is (.)

14       konkreettisesti jossain   on minkälaista se on,
         concrete-ADV    somewhere be how         it be
         concretely somewhere how it is

15 Ere:  nii että vähän opiskeluaki (.) siinä (.) sivussa
         yea so a bit studying (.) there (.) on the side

16 SW2:  nii,
         yea

17 SW1:  °mm°

18       (1.0)
```

Ere suggests that the participants make a visit to the employment office (lines 1–3). Yet, given that the proposal is produced in the context of planning the autumn season's program, the meaning of the proposal may not be entirely transparent to the other participants. And, indeed, after a silence (line 4), a support worker (SW1) asks for a clarification of the proposal, while offering one possible interpretation of its content (lines 5–7). Ere does not verify SW1's interpretation but nonetheless provides some clarification of his previous turn (lines 8–10). A relatively long silence ensues (line 11), after which the other support worker (SW2) provides an interpretation of what Ere has possibly been up to (lines 12–14), depicting his line of action as an expression of a "wish" (line 12). This is followed by Ere accounting for his action with reference to a possibility of "studying" (line 15). The responses by the two support workers are minimal (lines 16–17), although later in the episode they nevertheless end up writing Ere's idea down (not shown in the transcript).

In Extract 3, the two support workers clearly display interest in Ere's proposal. The use of the singular personal pronoun *sä* "you" in the support worker responses (lines 5 and 12) highlights their willingness to understand what Ere is specifically after. Simultaneously, however, the support workers' responses refrain from validating Ere's right to invite the whole group in decision-making about his idea. There are two aspects to this. First, the support workers' questions and candidate interpretations convey that Ere alone is accountable for clarifying his idea (see Helmer & Zinken, 2019), which leaves little room for others to contribute to the unfolding of interaction. Second, by framing Ere's action as an expression of individual wish, its status as a proposal that calls for joint deliberation of the group is undermined. Hence, the idea is not of the kind that should be given much space in the participants' interactional agenda.

Extract 4 represents a case in which the support workers' orientation may be placed somewhere *between other-orientation and self-orientation*. Here, the participants are planning the program for the spring season. At the beginning of the extract, a support worker (SW1) suggests a schedule for certain topics to be discussed in the group (lines 1–3), while her colleague (SW2) receives these ideas with tentative agreement (line 4). Thereafter, a client, Tua, produces a nominal utterance *työn mielekkyys* "sensibleness of work" (line 5), whose status as action is not very clear. In the context of the ongoing activity, however, her utterance can be understood as a proposal for a specific group discussion topic. However, the support workers do not react to Tua's utterance but instead, continue their previous discussion (lines 6–8). Thereafter, Tua produces another, extended turn, in which the status of her action as a proposal becomes clearer than before (lines 10–11).

Extract 4

```
01 SW1: olisko sit sen jälkeisel viikolla aiheena
        would we then next week have as a topic

02      sit toi että (.) palkkaus ja etuudet
        then that (.) wages and benefits

03      siirtymätyön palkkaus   ja [etuudet, ]
        transitional work wages and [benefits,]

04 SW2:                            [mm       ] vaikka.
                                   [mm       ] possibly.

05 Tua: työn mielekkyys.
        work-GEN sensibleness
        sensibleness of work

06 SW1: vai kerkeeks sen tohon samaan ton mitä on
        or can we make it in that same (slot) what is

07      siirtymätyö       (.) ei vält[tämättä,] ((writing))
        transitional work (.) not nec[essarily]

08 SW2:                             [ei vältt]is,
                                    [not nece]ssarily,

09      (0.4)

10 Tua: (työ) (.) työn     mielekkyys   olis     kans
        work      wokr-GEN sensibleness be-COND also
        (work) (.) the sensibleness of work would also be

11      semmonen (---) tykkää tehä (--) ja  ehkä    mä (--)
        sort.of        like   do-INF    and perhaps SG1
        a sort of (---) like to do (--) and perhaps I (--)

12 SW2: mitä siitä  vois
        what it-PAR could
        what could be (made) of it
```

13 Eki: (---) viittaa työn mielekkyyteen myös
(---) refers to the sensibleness of work also the

14 työn määrä (---) (samanlainen) (---)
amount of work (---) (similar) (---)

15 SW2: millä,
what-ADE
in what

16 Eki: (---)

17 SW2: millä tavalla me sitä, (1.2) käytäis
what-ADE manner-ADE PL1 it-PAR go-PASS-COND
how would we, (1.2) go

18 läpi, (1.0) me tehtiin <po:rtaita> niit
through PL1 do-PST-PASS stair-PL-PAR they-PAR
through it, (1.0) we did <strai:rs> those

19 itsearviointi- (0.7) °juttuja (0.2) sillon
self.evaluation- thing-PL-PAR then
self evaluation (0.7) °things° (0.2) then

20 viime (.) vuonna° (1.5) °oisko joku
last year-ESS be-COND-Q some
last (.) year° (1.5) would there be some

21 [muu° (.) muunlainen tapa toimia]
other other.kind.of manner act-INF
[other° (.) way to do it]

22 Eki: [(---)] mä
[(---)] I

23 löysin tämmösen (---) ((shows a paper))
found this kind of (---)

24 Mio: (--) työn määrä (-) tosi kaukaisia asioita mulle
(--) the amount of work (-) very remote things to me

The second version of Tua's proposal (lines 10–11) receives attention from the support workers. SW2 responds by asking "what could be [made] of it" (line 12). In response to SW2, a client, Eki, points out that the sensibleness of work is also related to the "amount of work" (lines 13–14). Thereafter, maintaining her previous line of action, SW2 repeats her question in a more elaborate form (lines 15, 17–21), referring to the ways in which such topics were discussed last year and asking whether this time there would be "some other way to do it" (lines 20–21). Thereafter. Eki takes up a paper that he shows to the other participants (lines 22–23) and comments on the topic (line 24).

As in Extract 3, the support worker reacts to the client's proposal by asking questions, thus displaying *other-orientation*. However, unlike in Extract 3, here the support worker's questions are not only targeted at the client, but at the whole group. Instead of using the second-person singular pronoun "you," the support worker uses the first-person plural pronoun "we" (lines 17–18), which encompasses the whole group, including the support worker herself, and thus conveys an element of *self-orientation*, too. Thus, instead of treating the proposer as accountable for being able to justify and clarify her proposal, the outcome of the proposal—including judgments about its feasibility and reasonability—is placed in the hands of the whole group. As can be seen in several clients later contributing to the conversation, this move indeed served as an effective way to encourage client participation.

Finally, Extract 5 represents an instance of *self-orientation* in the support workers' responses to client proposals. Here, the group has been discussing transitional work—a Clubhouse-created program offering employment opportunities for mental health clients (Valkeapää, Tanaka, Lindholm, Weiste, & Stevanovic, 2019). Line 1 shows the end of an explanation turn by one of the support workers (SW1), who has described the generic nature of the transitional work tasks: after the working period of one client, another client should be able to continue with the same job description. Thereafter, a client, Tia, suggests that those interested in the transitional work could visit the relevant workplaces to familiarize themselves with the workplace requirements (lines 2–5).

Extract 5

```
01 SW1: siihen aina uusi ihminen sitten saada.
        to get always a new person to that (job)

02 Tia: ja  sehän  tota niin niin ni  sehän vois   olla
        and it-CLI P    P    P    P it-CLI could be-INF
        and it is certainly so erm it could certainly be

03      niinki sit että se työ- ois     tiedossa se paikka
        P-CLI  P   CP   it work be-COND known    it place
        like that too that (when) that workplace is known

04      nii (.) ninku kävis   vähän ite  tutustumassa
        P       P     go-COND a.bit self familiarize-INF-INE
        so (.) like one would go oneself to get to

05      siihe   vaikka esimerkiks,
        into.it P       for.example
        know it a bit say for example

06 SW1: nääkin   ois kivoja.
        these-CLI be-COND nice-PL-PAR
        these would also be nice

07 SW2: ja  tosta    tulee mulla   Tia  heti nyt mieleen
        and that-ELA come  SG1-ADE Name just now mind-ILL
        and from that Tia I now became immediately

08      et niinki villi ajatus  et me  voitas    ehkä
        CP P-CLI  wild  thought CP PL1 could-PASS perhaps
        such a wild idea that we could perhaps

09      vähän puhua    että ku kaupungissaki on
        a.bit speak-INF CP   P  city-INE-CLI  be
        a bit discuss since in the city there are also

10      monenlaisia   paikkoja     ja  muita        niin
        various-PL-PAR place-PL-PAR and other-PL-PAR P
        various places and else so (one could)
```

```
11        kysästä et oisko      siellä joku semmonen mihin
          ask-INF CP be-COND-Q there  some sort.if  in.where
          ask if there would be something where

12        me  päästäs        vaik kattoon     tai tutustuu
          PL1 get-PASS-COND P    see-INF-ILL or  get.to.know
          we could get say to see or get to know

13        mitä se työ  ninku kon- oikeesti on siellä.
          what it work P          real-ADV be there
          what that work like concr- really is there

14 SW1:   niin kyllä.
          yeah yes.

15 Tia:   joo,
          yea,

16 SW2:   en uskalla luvata että päästään mihinkään
          I don't dare to promise that we get anywhere

17        mutta voidaanhan me tosiaan (---)
          but certainly we could (---)

18 Ava:   se ois ihan hyvä.
          it would be pretty good

19 Tia:   niin se tutustuminen olis
          yeah that getting to know (the place) would be

20        minusta kyllä aika tärkeetä
          in my opinion surely quite important
```

Tia's proposal (lines 2–5) is followed by SW1's positive evaluation turn, whose referent is however somewhat unclear (note the plural forms in line 6). Thereafter, her colleague (SW2) produces a lengthy proposal turn (lines 7–13). While the idea is presented as being based on Tia's previous proposal (see lines 7–8), the idea is nonetheless framed as an individual proposal by SW2 herself—and, furthermore, as an unconventional one (note the word *villi* "wild," line 8). SW1 and Tia receive SW2's proposal with agreement tokens (lines 14–15), after which SW2 expresses reservations about whether her idea could indeed be realized (lines

16–17). In response to that, Ava offers a positive evaluation of SW2's idea (line 18). Finally, Tia produces a turn in which she not only agrees with the idea but also displays independence toward it (lines 19–20). The turn-initial particle *niin* "yeah" (line 19) invokes the speaker's prior epistemic access to the content of the proposal (Sorjonen, 2001), while the phrase "in my opinion" (line 20) avoids treating the idea as anything but the speaker's own creation. In so doing, Tia reclaims ownership of the idea, in the face of the support worker's proposal being almost identical to hers.

Thus, instead of focusing on trying to understand the details of, and the reasoning behind, the client's proposal, the support worker only acknowledges it as an inspiration for a proposal of her own. In so doing, similar to Extract 4, she indirectly validates the relevance of the client's proposal by de facto giving it space in the participants' interactional agenda. However, unlike in Extract 4, where the support worker asked questions to invite the whole group to engage in joint deliberation about the content of the proposal, here, the support worker herself demonstrates such deliberation (note the first-person singular pronoun "I" in line 7). As we can see in the subsequent unfolding of the sequence, paradoxically, this support worker's move served as an effective way to encourage further client participation.

Conclusions

In this chapter, we asked how support workers in rehabilitation group meetings at the Clubhouse respond to client proposals, thus opening and closing opportunities for the other clients to participate in the ongoing decision-making. To increase understanding of the complexity of the phenomenon at hand, we described two dilemmas that the support workers face when seeking to take the clients' proposals "seriously."

The first dilemma concerned the meeting's *agenda*. With reference to Extracts 1–2 we pointed to a sufficiently slow progression of decision-making as being a prerequisite for collective participation in a group. This prerequisite, however, puts proposers in a vulnerable position: to slow down decision-making and to encourage collective participation, support workers may need to refrain from providing substantial approval for the clients' proposals. Drawing on Goffman (1959, 1967), it has been argued elsewhere that "one aspect by which one's self is particularly vulnerable to interaction is one's right to determine action" (Stevanovic, 2018, p. 6). While the mere act of making a proposal involves a claim of such a right in terms of future actions or events, what is particularly at stake in a group meeting is the proposer's right to determine the participants' actions *now*. Considering the slow pace in which decisions may be made by a group, a single proposal may influence the meeting's agenda for a relatively long time period. It is thus especially during group decision-making when offering proposers recognition for their interactional contributions would be needed.

The other dilemma had to do with the distribution of *agency*. Inspired by Enfield (2011), we considered two questions as central in this regard: (1) who is accountable for the feasibility and reasonability of the proposal and (2) who is accountable for its relevance to the whole group. Here, our analysis highlighted a tension between focusing on the client as the originator of the proposal and avoiding treating him or her alone as being accountable for it. From this perspective, we described the paradoxical consequences that the support workers' self vs. other-orientation, as exhibited in their responses, had for the participation dynamics of the group. Extract 3 demonstrated how other-orientation—the use of the second-person singular pronoun "you" in questions—was associated with holding the client alone accountable for clarifying the content of the proposal. Thereby, the proposed idea was also framed as an individual wish of the client, which does not make relevant group decision-making. Extract 4 exemplified an orientation somewhere between other- vs. self-orientation. The support worker's use of the first-person plural pronoun "we," again in a question, called for everybody to consider how the suggested idea could be realized. Such responses were seen to highlight the relevance of the proposal for the whole group and circumvent the proposer's individual accountability for it.

Finally, Extract 5 represented an instance of self-orientation, which was reflected in the support worker's use of the first-person singular pronoun "I" in a proposal that was produced as a response to a client proposal of almost identical content. The response thus highlighted the support worker's full agency in relation to the suggested idea. While such interactional moves may not respect the clients' ownership of their ideas, these support worker responses led to a relatively high level of participation in the group. One possible explanation of this finding is that the support worker's own demonstration of deliberation affects the collective participation dynamics in a way parallel to what Tannen (2005) has referred to as "high-involvement" interaction style. In this style, the participants' primary concern is not "to make it comfortable and convenient for others to express their ideas, but rather to be free and spontaneous with reactions" (Tannen, 2005, p. 138). Based on the insights of Tannen, Svennevig (2014) examined conversations between strangers and argued that shifts to high-involvement style and self-oriented turns indicate and encourage emotional closeness and taken-for-grantedness of mutual concern. It is thus possible that the support workers in our data, through their self-oriented responses to client proposals, succeeded in establishing such a high-involvement interactional environment.

With this chapter, we sought to contribute to a deeper understanding of joint decision-making in a group. While the dilemmas of agenda and agency described here are presumably relevant to any group decision-making situation, in the context of mental health clients, additional sensitivity to these concerns may be needed. For example, when it comes to the management of the tension between individual recognition and group decision-making, support workers' heightened sensitivity to the tension may help them to calibrate their responsive behaviors to find the locally appropriate balance between individual and collective well-being (Seligman & Csikszentmihalyi, 2000). In response to routine proposals, individual recognition for the proposer could perhaps be compromised in favor of increasing the level of group participation. In contrast, in response to more unconventional or delicate proposals, where a lack of recognition could lead to embarrassment, group participation could be compromised in favor of individual recognition.

Against some mundane expectations of what constitutes polite behavior, our data analysis also highlighted the problematic nature of other-orientation. The *other-oriented* support worker responses to client proposals seem to invoke client accountability in ways that, besides possibly threatening the client's face (Goffman, 1967), may also exclude others from decision-making. Instead, and paradoxically, the support workers' *self-oriented* responses seem to open up a more relaxed way for client participation. Ultimately, it is a free and safe interactional atmosphere that everyone seeking to contribute to joint decision-making desires and the creation of such an atmosphere may be even more important among participants with mental illness.

References

Angouri, J., & Marra, M. (2011). Corporate meetings as genre: A study of the role of the chair in corporate meeting talk. *Text & Talk, 30*(6), 615–636.

Atkinson, J. M., & Drew, P. (1979). *Order in court: The organisation of verbal interaction in judicial settings*. London, UK: Macmillan.

Boden, D. (1994). *The business of talk: Organizations in action*. Cambridge: Polity Press.

Enfield, N. (2011). Sources of asymmetry in human interaction: Enchrony, status, knowledge and agency. In T. Stivers, L. Mondada, & J. Steensig (Eds.), *The morality of knowledge in conversation* (pp. 285–312). Cambridge: Cambridge University Press.

Garfinkel, H. (1967). *Studies in ethnomethodology*. Englewood Cliffs, NJ: Prentice-Hall.

Goffman, E. (1959). *The presentation of self in everyday life*. Woodstock: Overlook Press.

Goffman, E. (1967). *Interaction ritual*. Garden City: Anchor Books.

Goffman, E. (1981). *Forms of talk*. Oxford: Basil Blackwell.

Greatbatch, D. (1988). A turn-taking system for British news interviews. *Language in Society, 17*(3), 401–430.

Helmer, H., & Zinken, J. (2019). *Das heißt* ("That means") for formulations and *Du meinst* ("You mean") for repair? Interpretations of prior speakers' turns in German. *Research on Language and Social Interaction, 52*(2), 159–176.

Kendall, S. (1993). Do health visitors promote client participation? An analysis of the health visitor–client interaction. *Journal of Clinical Nursing, 2*(2), 103–109.

Lukes, S. (1974). *Power: A radical view*. London: Macmillan.

Mehan, H. (1979). *Learning lessons: Social organisation on the classroom*. Cambridge, MA: Harvard University Press.

Schegloff, E. A. (2007). *Sequence organization in interaction: A primer in conversation analysis*. Cambridge: Cambridge University Press.
Seligman, M. E. P., & Csikszentmihalyi, M. (2000). Positive psychology: An introduction. *American Psychologist, 55*(1), 5–14.
Sorjonen, M.-L. (2001). *Responding in conversation: A study of response particles in Finnish*. Amsterdam, NL: Benjamins.
Stevanovic, M. (2012). Establishing joint decisions in a dyad. *Discourse Studies, 14*(6), 779–803.
Stevanovic, M. (2013). Constructing a proposal as a thought: A way to manage problems in the initiation of joint decision-making in Finnish workplace interaction. *Pragmatics, 23*(3), 519–544.
Stevanovic, M. (2015). Displays of uncertainty and proximal deontic claims: The case of proposal sequences. *Journal of Pragmatics, 78*, 84–97.
Stevanovic, M. (2018). Social deontics: A nano-level approach to human power play. *Journal for the Theory of Social Behaviour, 48*(3), 369–389.
Stevanovic, M., & Peräkylä, A. (2012). Deontic authority in interaction: The right to announce, propose and decide. *Research on Language and Social Interaction, 45*(3), 297–321.
Stevanovic, M., & Weiste, E. (2017). Conversation analytic data session as a pedagogical institution. *Learning, Culture, and Social Interaction, 15*, 1–17.
Svennevig, J. (2014). Direct and indirect self-presentation in first conversations. *Journal of Language and Social Psychology, 33*(3), 302–327.
Tannen, D. (2005). *Conversational style: Analyzing talk among friends*. New York: Oxford University Press.
Valkeapää, T., Tanaka, K., Lindholm, C., Weiste, E., & Stevanovic, M. (2019). Interaction, ideology, and practice in mental health rehabilitation. *Journal of Psychosocial Rehabilitation and Mental Health, 6*(1), 9–23.

7

Engaging with Clients' Requests for Medication Changes in Psychiatry

Galina B. Bolden, Alexa Hepburn, and Beth Angell

Negotiating Treatment Decisions in Psychiatry

In psychiatry, as in other medical fields, practitioners are encouraged to adopt a patient-centered approach that emphasizes the sharing of decisions with their clients (Angell, Matthews, Stanhope, & Rowe, 2015; Corrigan et al., 2012; Drake & Deegan, 2009). At the same time, psychiatrists operate under an institutional responsibility to prescribe medications to clients who may be mandated to treatment or at risk of harm to self or

G. B. Bolden (✉) · A. Hepburn
Department of Communication, Rutgers University,
New Brunswick, NJ, USA
e-mail: gbolden@comminfo.rutgers.edu

A. Hepburn
e-mail: alexa.hepburn@rutgers.edu

B. Angell
School of Social Work, Virginia Commonwealth University,
Richmond, VA, USA
e-mail: keangell@vcu.edu

C. Lindholm et al. (eds.), *Joint Decision Making in Mental Health*,
The Language of Mental Health, https://doi.org/10.1007/978-3-030-43531-8_7

others when not under treatment. The negotiation of treatment decisions in chronic psychiatric care is particularly delicate since clients might not possess awareness of their illness and may resist taking the medications, putting psychiatrists in the position of persuading clients to accept and adhere to the treatment (Carter, 2003; Olfson, Marcus, Wilk, & West, 2006). However, this exercise of clinician authority does not mean that decisions are necessarily made unilaterally and that clients are passive recipients of clinicians' proposals.

Research into psychiatric interactions conducted in the conversation analytic tradition (Sidnell & Stivers, 2013) has brought to light some interactional practices involved in negotiating and agreeing on a treatment plan (Land, Parry, & Seymour, 2017). The analysis of actual recorded psychiatric consultations has shown that psychiatrists commonly present their treatment decisions as shared by designing their recommendations in ways that convey a degree of patient agency, formatting them as, for example, proposals, suggestions, and offers (Bolden & Angell, 2017; Thompson & McCabe, 2017). At the same time, psychiatrists tend to steer the treatment discussion toward a particular outcome. For example, psychiatrists may apply pressure on their clients by eliciting a commitment from them or direct them toward a particular treatment by marking it as a best option (Quirk, Chaplin, Lelliott, & Seale, 2012). Psychiatrists may also design their recommendations so as to fit the client's perspective (Kushida & Yamakawa, 2015) and address the client's concerns (Angell & Bolden, 2015, 2016; Bolden & Angell, 2017). Additionally, they may justify and account for their recommendations in ways that draw on their medical authority (Angell & Bolden, 2015, 2016; Bolden & Angell, 2017). While much of this research has focused on the communicative work psychiatrists do to promote their treatment decisions, recent studies have also begun to explore communicative practices clients use to advocate for particular medication regimens (Bolden, Angell, & Hepburn, 2019; Kushida, Hiramoto, & Yamakawa, 2016).

In our analysis of psychiatric consultations with clients who have severe mental illnesses (schizophrenia, bipolar disorders, etc.), we have examined the organization of consultations that have an explicit institutional agenda as "medication check" appointments (Angell & Bolden, 2015, 2016; Bolden & Angell, 2017; Bolden, Angell, & Hepburn, 2019).

In our dataset (see the discussion of the setting below), a routine medication check appointment unfolds quite similarly to other medical visits (Robinson, 2003), especially those dealing with chronic illnesses (Bolden & Angell, 2017; Koenig, Wingard, Sabee, Olsher, & Vandergriff, 2014). While other topics are typically discussed (such as the client's living arrangements and family relationships), the medical agenda is evident throughout the visit. Thus, following the opening of the visit, the initial phase of the appointment is *data gathering*, during which the psychiatrist asks a series of probing questions into how the client is feeling, thinking, sleeping, managing social relationships, etc. The clients in this dataset have had a psychiatric diagnosis for a long time, so the issue is not whether they have a particular psychiatric condition but how well the condition is being managed by the current medications. These questions—not unlike history taking in other kinds of medical interactions (Boyd & Heritage, 2006)—serve to evaluate how well the medications are working, both therapeutically to control the client's psychiatric symptoms and in terms of the harmful side effects. Next, the psychiatrist offers an *assessment* of the client's *current clinical status*. Subsequently, possible changes in the *treatment* plan—that is, whether (and how) to modify doses or types of medication the client takes—may be discussed extensively (Bolden & Angell, 2017).

As we have shown in prior work (Bolden et al., 2019), when clients solicit medication changes, they commonly do so at the point where the psychiatrist begins the move into the business of the visit after the opening. Additionally, clients may launch the topic of medication change later in the visit, sometimes quite disjunctively, taking advantage of other activity transitions during the data-gathering phase.

In order to solicit a medication change, clients have been found to deploy the following practices (Bolden et al., 2019). First, they may report a physical problem that is hearable as a medication side effect (such as drowsiness, drooling, or tremor), with or without attributing the problem to a particular medication. Second, they may explicitly request a medication change (e.g., "I was wondering if you could take it away"). Additionally, they may demand a change (e.g., "I want my meds lowered"). By using one of these solicitation practices, the client puts pressure on the psychiatrist to respond in a particular way—for example, to either offer a solution to the reported problem and/or to accept (or reject) the client's request for a medication adjustment. In this chapter, we explore how, exactly, the psychiatrist engages with clients' solicitation of a medication change.

Building on this line of research, the present chapter sheds further light on how psychiatrists engage with clients' requests, and how psychiatrists and clients come to an agreement about a treatment plan. We analyze how medication decisions unfold when clients advocate for their treatment preferences (Bolden et al., 2019). Our focus is on how the psychiatrist responds to clients' requests for changes in their medication regimen, for example, requests to eliminate or lower dosages of psychotropic medications or to prescribe a new medication. Our analysis presents the two alternative interactional trajectories clients' requests for medication changes may engender: a serious engagement with the request and its outright dismissal. We will show that, in both scenarios, the psychiatrist works to validate the clients' participation in their care by engagement with clients' expressed preferences.

Research Questions

In this chapter, we investigate the psychiatrist's uptake to clients' requests for changes in their medication. We address the following research questions:

- When the psychiatrist either engages or dismisses clients' requests for medication changes, what interactional trajectories does this engagement engender?
- What interactional practices are deployed by the psychiatrist to encourage client participation in treatment decisions following their requests?

Setting and Data

This study examines psychiatrist–client interactions in the context of a comprehensive treatment service known as assertive community treatment (or ACT). ACT programs provide intensive community-based support via an interdisciplinary treatment team, frequently including social workers, nurses, psychologists, and a psychiatrist. Treatment plans are tailored to client needs, incorporating medication management, training in everyday life tasks, supportive psychotherapy, and assistance with gaining disability benefits and housing. A hallmark of the model is the assertiveness of efforts to offer services to clients, even if they exhibit reluctance or ambivalence about treatment. ACT services include the prescription and ongoing (daily, if necessary) monitoring and delivery of psychiatric medications, ensuring that clients follow prescribed medication regimens. Our analysis focuses on how psychiatrists and clients negotiate ongoing changes in medication type and dose during regularly scheduled consultations, commonly referred to as "medication check" appointments (see also Angell & Bolden, 2015, 2016; Bolden & Angell, 2017; Bolden et al., 2019).

Within the ACT model, medications are a cornerstone of treatment and are provided via a long-term relationship with a psychiatrist, who is often employed directly by the program. Psychiatric appointments are scheduled at regular intervals as part of the program's comprehensive medication support function, which frequently includes procurement and daily delivery of medications to clients in addition to prescribing and monitoring activities (Allness & Knoedler, 2003). While the explicit purpose of these appointments is medication management, psychiatrists working within ACT tend to adopt a generalist orientation to treatment that involves discussing lifestyle issues (such as living arrangements, family relationships, and work activities) in addition to the medication regimen. Because of the variable course of serious mental disorders, psychiatric appointments serve to monitor the client's stability and responses to medication, and to make adjustments to the medications in order to optimize the client's capacity to cope with the illness and pursue personally determined psychosocial goals.

The data for this study come from audio-recordings of medication check appointments collected in 2009–2010 in an established ACT program in a mid-sized city in the United States. We examined 36 audio-recorded interactions between a team psychiatrist and her clients (sometimes with a case manager present), each lasting between 15 and 45 minutes. In all of the recorded visits, the clients have been on various psychotropic medications for several years, and, as a result, have accumulated a substantial amount of knowledge about their functioning and side effects. All names and other identifiers on the transcripts are pseudonyms. Informed consent to audio-record and use collected data for research purposes was obtained from all participants.

The study uses the methodology of conversation analysis, which examines the interactional practices participants use to carry out courses of action through a close analysis of naturally occurring interactions (Sidnell & Stivers, 2013). For this study, the audio-recorded consultations were transcribed following conversation analytic transcription conventions (Hepburn & Bolden, 2017). A collection of cases in which clients may be seen as soliciting (directly or implicitly) a medication adjustment has been analyzed for this study (27 in total, from 15 consultations in which medication adjustment solicitations were found). The data extracts included in the chapter are drawn from two consultations and were selected for their clarity in representing the target interactional practices.

Building Consensus Following Clients' Requests for Medication Changes

A client's request for a medication change typically engenders a series of questions from the psychiatrist—an expansive insert sequence designed to interrogate the client's grounds for the request before a response to the request is provided (Schegloff, 2007). In this section, we illustrate this trajectory by analyzing how one such request (to be taken off a psychotropic medication) unfolds through a series of extracts from one consultation. We show that even though the psychiatrist ultimately rejects the client's request, this decision is presented as neither unilateral nor in conflict with the client's preferences. Rather, the psychiatrist validates the grounds for the client's request, and presents her treatment plan (to lower the medication in question) as being in line with what the client had requested.

Interrogating Grounds for the Client's Request

Extract 1a is taken from the very beginning of the visit. The psychiatrist has just explained that the appointment is to see how things are going in light of recent medication changes (data not shown). In line 1, the psychiatrist solicits an update from the client with *what's ↑up*, a typical question format for soliciting "chronic-routine" patient concerns (Robinson, 2006). This question creates an opportunity for the client to raise his medication problems. In line 2, the client begins to report a problem with one of his medications, Geodon, and subsequently explicitly requests to discontinue the medication (see Bolden et al., 2019 for a discussion of this segment).

Extract 1a

```
01 P: So what's ↑up
02 C: Uh::: we:ll, Geodon's the problem now.=That's eh-
03    that's the one that'sh:: like the sedation of it
04    whatever it is¿ .hhh I keep getting a dro:wsi=
05    =sleepiness feelin',
06    (1.0)
07 C: .hh Uh::: (.) t! I was wonderin' if you could take
08    it awa:y, an' (.) make #e-um:: .hhhh li:ke uh::
09    whatever med I'm on make it more higher or something¿
10    (.)
11 C: to-to replace that or something¿
12 P: Oka:y,
13 C: Cuz' that's the pro:blem=I seem like (0.2)
14    I'm ge- jus coming back to that dro:wsy
15    sleepiness feeling.
16 P: Ok[ay.
17 C:   [that I- that I used to get back the:n, .h
18 P: So is it coming ba:ck, or has it been there
19    all alo::ng.
```

The client takes several medications, some of which may cause drowsiness, so his claim (in line 2) that *Geodon's the problem* is very strong and thus potentially suspicious. The client immediately extends his turn to formulate a possible connection between Geodon and drowsiness. This extension is epistemically downgraded (with *whatever it is*), and in the course of the extended report, the client replaces more technical terms *sedation* and *drowsiness* with a less technical one *sleepiness feeling* (line 5), thus displaying an orientation to encroaching onto the psychiatrist's professional expertise (Kitzinger & Mandelbaum, 2013). Following this problem presentation, there is a one-second gap (line 6) where an uptake from the psychiatrist is due. This lack of uptake may be hearable as delegitimizing the reported problem. In line 7, the client extends his turn further, now articulating an explicit request to discontinue Geodon. The request is designed in the *I was wondering* format, which is a way to convey the client's low entitlement to making the request and the high contingency of the requested outcome (Curl & Drew, 2008), and underscores the delicacy of the action. In lines 8–9, the client extends the request with the proposal to raise another medication he is taking. This is again produced quite tentatively (*whatever med I'm on*; *more higher or something*; *replace that or something*), which works to preserve the psychiatrist's expertise and downgrade the client's epistemic authority. At the same time, by offering an alternative, the client removes a possible hearing of his request as asking to be off his medications entirely, thus working to present himself as a "good patient" who understands the need for medications (Bolden et al., 2019).

Our primary interest here is in the psychiatrist's uptake to the client's request. In lines 18–19, the psychiatrist launches an insert sequence designed to assess the validity of the request (Schegloff, 2007). Note that the psychiatrist builds her question to display responsiveness to the client's problem formulation. She picks up on the concerns the client brought up (the *dro:wsy sleepiness feeling … coming ba:ck*; lines 14–15, 19), reusing the client's own formulation (*coming ba:ck*) in her interrogative so as to enact client-attentiveness (Angell & Bolden, 2015). Additionally, by prefacing the question with *so*, the psychiatrist presents her inquiry as arising out of the client's concerns

(Bolden, 2009; Heritage & Watson, 1979). This question begins a lengthy interrogative series (cf. Zimmerman, 1984) in which the psychiatrist investigates the current state of the client's health and how it might have been impacted by this and the other medications he is taking. In doing so, the psychiatrist engages with and takes seriously the grounds for the client's request (to take him off Geodon), thereby validating the client's right to make the request (see also Chapter 6 in this volume).

Following three-and-half minutes of this investigation, the psychiatrist summarizes her assessment with the following diagnostic upshot (lines 25–26):

Extract 1b

```
20 P: =Uhm (.) but you're still sleepin' #good.
21    [which    is    really    ]positive.#
22 C: [I'm still sleeping good]
23 P:  Okay. .hh Uh:m (0.5) okay.
24    (0.2)
25 P: .hh Well it does sound (.) kinda like the
26    Geodon's the culprit. doesn't it.
27 C: Yeah[:.
```

Several features of this diagnostic upshot (lines 25–26) stand out. First, it is designed to agree with and confirm the client's own diagnostic assessment that Geodon is responsible for drowsiness (lines 2–5 in Extract 1a). Second, it is built with an emphasis on *does*, which, on the one hand, claims the psychiatrist's primary rights to make this diagnostic assessment (Stivers, 2005) and, on the other hand, presents this conclusion as contrastive with the psychiatrist's prior understanding or expectation (Raymond, 2017). Third, the psychiatrist presents her diagnostic conclusion as grounded in what the client has reported to her by using the evidential verb *sound* (line 25). The use of the evidential (as well as the modifier *kinda*) downgrades the certainty of the diagnosis (Peräkylä, 1998). Finally, the psychiatrist extends her turn constructional unit (Sacks, Schegloff, & Jefferson, 1974) with the tag question (*doesn't it.*; line 26), thereby presenting this as a shared understanding and inviting the client to confirm it (which he does in line 27) (Heritage & Raymond, 2005). In other words, the psychiatrist designs her diagnostic upshot in ways that attribute to the client the role of a co-diagnostician—somebody who is capable of observing his symptoms and drawing conclusions from them. This validates the client's involvement in the treatment decision (cf. Land, Parry, & Seymour, 2017).

Proposing and Justifying a Treatment Change

Thirty-five seconds later, following further justification involving running through different medications the client is taking and their side effects, the psychiatrist produces her treatment recommendation—to reduce the dosage of Geodon:

Extract 1c

```
28 P: [okay.    ] Good.
29     (.)
30 P: .hh Uhm (0.5) so I think (0.5) we've been gradually
31    working to reduce the Geodon,
32     (.)
33 P: an' it's go:in' okay,
34     (.)
35 P: y'[know,
36 C:    [mm hmm,
37 P: .h uh::m (0.2) so it makes sense we could reduce it
38    some more.
39    (0.2)
40 P: [°ya know°
41 C: [Okay
42 P: .h An' it- Let's check about ho:w other stuff's going
43    on too. Just to make su::r:e that (.) everything's
44    goin' okay? ↑before we reduce it?
45 C: [(°°Mm mm°°)
46 P: ['T sounds like it. but .hh we'll go kinda though
47    (0.5) y'know the stuff where we've asked you about
48    before,
49    (.)
50 P: like uh:m your sleep is good, you told me tha:t,
```

In lines 30–37, the psychiatrist formulates independent grounds for the treatment change, thus presenting the suggested reduction not as a simple acquiescence to the client's request but as a logical continuation of their ongoing treatment plan (*makes sense*; line 37). Note that the recommendation to reduce Geodon does not grant the client's request, which was to take him off this medication entirely. Yet, by first presenting herself as being in agreement with the client (about Geodon being *the culprit* in line 26), the proposed alternative treatment plan (to reduce Geodon) is brought off as being in line with what the client had requested.

The psychiatrist presents the treatment plan as somewhat tentative (*could reduce*; line 37). Additionally, by using the collective person reference *we* (rather than *I* in line 37) she may be including the client in the decision-making process—though there are other team members involved in the client's care, whom she is also including here (Bolden & Angell, 2017). The ambiguity about whether the client is part of the *we* might be a designed one, casting the decision as a collaborative activity that potentially includes the client (Angell & Bolden, 2016; Bolden & Angell, 2017).

In line 42, the psychiatrist reopens the data-gathering phase of the visit in order to get a more complete picture of the client's current clinical status. The *Let's check* formulation enrolls the client into this additional investigation. In line 44, the psychiatrist recasts her prior decision to reduce Geodon as conditional on the results of this investigation. During the subsequent talk (not shown), the client again maintains that Geodon is the cause of his drowsiness problem.

In Extract 1d (which takes place three minutes later), the psychiatrist reintroduces the client's original request (to *take away* the Geodon), by bringing up the associated risks involved (lines 51–54). In this way, the psychiatrist justifies her decision to reduce, rather than eliminate, the drug—that is, justifies her rejection of the client's request.

Extract 1d

```
51 P: Good. .h So the risk is we take the Geodon away,
52    is that (.) for some reason it's still not enou:gh,
53    the Seroquel is still not enou:gh, an' you might
54    have some change in your slee:p, #or:# .hh start
55    that irritable feelin' again, #or something like
56    that. s[o#
57 C:        [Well I'd- I'm getting into ma=my personal
58    opinion,
59    (0.2)
60 C: .h I think it will wo:rk if you took it away¿
61    Jus me just me personally sayin' how it's been
62    working with me,
63 P: Mm hm?
64 C: working on th'insi:de me, 'n' thinkin I think if
65    you took it away, (0.2) .hhh it wouldn't- it wouldn't
66    like affect anythi:ng, or make- or cha:nge anythi:ng,
67 P: °°mm hm°°
68 C: I jus jus me persona<That's just my personal=
69 P: =We:ll, (.) I mean itch you:r body.
70    an' y[ou have (.)
71 C:      [yeah:
72 P: Y'know y[ou have a sense of things. like tha:t,
73 C:         [°yah°
74    y'know how it's affecting you better than (.)
75    I would.
76   (.)
77 P: Y'know in that way, so [.hh I just
78 C:                        [°Right°
79 P: need to tell you tha:t. cause I- we always tell
80    peo:ple (.) like the risks.  .hh Just in case
81    we have to rai:se the Seroquel.for some reason,
82    but (.) at this point we know ya so well:: (.)
83    y'know I think (0.2) .hh you an' John've been
84    communicatin' we::ll, an' so: if anything ha:ppens,
85    (0.5) we can jus (0.2) take care of it. 'n' (.)
86    y'know raise that do:se.
87 C: Righ[t.
88 P:     [So:. .hhhh uhm (0.5) t! (0.5) I think
89    it makes sense to- (.) to go do:wn agai:n, an-
90    (0.2) maybe to keep going do:wn?=instead of waiting
91    so lo:ng in betwee:n?=like we have been?
92 C: Mm hm.
```

In lines 57–58, following the psychiatrist's justification (for not discontinuing Geodon entirely), the client begins to put up a rather strong resistance to this position, presenting the objection as his *personal opinion* (lines 57–58) based on how it has been *working on th'insi:de me* (line 64). Here, the client clearly orients to the boundaries of both his own and the psychiatrist's epistemic authority—both in highlighting his personal experiences with the medications, to which the psychiatrist has no access ("epistemics of experience"; Heritage, 2013) and in downgrading the status of his position throughout: for example, *Jus me just me personally sayin'* (line 61), *I jus jus me persona* < *That's just my personal* (line 68).

In response, in lines 69–79, the psychiatrist validates his position by conceding that the client has epistemic authority over his own bodily experiences (Heritage, 2013). She then frames her prior reference to risks as something that is normatively done in this situation, using the institutional *we* (*we always tell peo:ple*; lines 79–81), thereby invoking her professional expertise (Angell & Bolden, 2016). The psychiatrist goes on to explain a contingency plan (to raise Seroquel; lines 80–85) and compliments the client's communication skills (lines 83–84). Finally, the psychiatrist reformulates the treatment recommendation upshot: to keep decreasing Geodon, possibly at a faster pace (lines 88–91). This treatment decision is again hedged in various ways (for example, with *I think* and *maybe*), and the rising intonation (line 91) appears to invite a response from the client.

Overall, this series of extracts presents a number of interactional practices through which the psychiatrist encourages the client to become an active participant in making decisions about his treatment. As we have seen, the psychiatrist validates the client's right to make the medication change request by launching an investigation into its grounds. She subsequently agrees with the client's grounds for the request (thereby validating his role as a co-diagnostician), and engages the client in reaching a compromise treatment plan. Thus, the psychiatrist works to balance her decisional authority with an orientation to patient involvement (Bolden & Angell, 2017).

An Alternative Path: Dismissing Clients' Requests for Medication Changes

In this section, we analyze a different path clients' requests for a medication change sometimes take: when the psychiatrist rejects the request without investigating the validity of the grounds on which it was made. By rejecting a request without interrogating its grounds, the psychiatrist conveys the stance that the request is baseless. In our data, such rejections are uncommon, but they occur in some situations. For instance: when a client requests a new medication that is treated as transparently inappropriate given the client's diagnosis; when the request occurs later in the consultation, after the client's clinical status has already been explored and a decision about treatment made; and/or when the request is deemed unwarranted for other reasons (e.g., due to the client's mental health history), as in the case discussed below. We will show that, even though the psychiatrist makes a unilateral decision to reject the client's request without investigating its grounds, she still works to cast the client's involvement in his treatment decision-making as valid.

Rejecting the Client's Request Without Investigation

Earlier in the visit from which this series of extracts is drawn, the client says that he is doing *terrible* (data not shown). Just prior to Extract 2a, the client and the psychiatrist have been discussing whether or not the client practices safe sex. In line 1, the psychiatrist transitions back to the business of the visit, and the client uses this as an opportunity to demand a medication change: *I wan' my meds lowered* (line 3). The demand format (rare in our data) presents the client as highly entitled to get his wish fulfilled (Bolden et al., 2019).

Extract 2a

```
P: So we got a liddle off topic the:re unless::_
   (1.7) u:m:
C: I wan' my meds lowered.
   (0.8)
C: 'S third time ya'll lowered mah meds for no reason.
   First time's: (0.5) back in two thousan 'n six when
   (.) .dhh Beth said (0.3) '↑oh he need 'is meds raised.'
   an just c's Beth said it ya'll raised my meds. .Hh (.)
   An' then second time was when I went to the hospital
   .hh when a dude call the p'lice on me (0.6) because he
   w- he was you- <he wasn' on the right medication.
   (0.8)
C: And uh: so he just decided the best way to get rid o'
   me .hh was de lie to the police and tell em dat I wanna
   kill 'im.
   (0.4)
P: Mhm:.
C: .dhh No matter how you look at it I did not wanna kill
   that ma:n. I knew he wun' doin no'hin' to: me,
   (.)
C: .hh Anyway 'e call'd th' police on me an > 'n then all
   of a sudden I godda< go to a hospital:, .hh Ya'll
   raised my meds fifteen milligrams fer that °shit°.
   (.)
P: Mhm=
C: =That's bull shit.
   (0.4)
C: An' then uh: (.) all'a sudden, (0.5) three months
   ago,=ya'll raised my meds again.=It's bull shit.
   (0.2)
P: .Hhh (.)
P: ↑Mm hmm::,=
C: =I wan' ma meds lowered.
   (0.5)
C: Back to ten milligram:s.
P: Oh Ro:[na:::ld_
C:       [(Ten milligrams) Yap,
P: Ten milligrams wadn't really helpin you much at ↑a::ll.
   #back th[en.#
C:          [Yes it wa:s:.
P: (Ah) Th't wasn't <↑my: recollection,>=
```

When the psychiatrist produces no uptake to the client's demand for a medication change (see the gap in line 4), the client begins to account for the demand (lines 5–29). Unlike Extract 1, where the client grounded his request for a medication change in harmful side effects, here the client narrates a series of prescription decisions, which has resulted, in his view, in an unjustifiably high dosage. The psychiatrist responds with only a minimal uptake throughout the telling (lines 17, 25), and a resistant continuer ↓*Mm hmm:*:, (line 32), where the client's telling is possibly complete and an action-relevant uptake is due (Schegloff, 1982). The client then reiterates his demand (*I wan' ma meds lowered.*), and (after no uptake in line 34) extends it to specify the dosage (*Back to ten milligram:s.*; line 35).

In line 36, rather than begin investigative questioning (as we saw in Extract 1a), the psychiatrist immediately rejects the client's more specific demand with a dismissive *Oh Ro:[na:::ld_*. This *oh*-prefaced, prosodically exaggerated address term response (see Hepburn & Potter, 2011; Heritage, 1998) seems to treat the client's demand as undeserving of a serious consideration. In lines 38–39, the psychiatrist justifies this rejection by claiming that the dosage the client wants was not therapeutic. The rest of the visit continues along these lines, with an open dispute about whether or not the client needs the medications.

Thus, in this visit, the decision (to keep the medications unchanged) is made unilaterally by the psychiatrist, without taking into consideration the client's wishes. However, throughout much of the rest of the visit, the psychiatrist works to convince the client that the decision is the right one for him, in an attempt to get him to accept it. While this is unsuccessful, and the client continues to resist the decision, the psychiatrist's continuous engagement in the debate with the client displays her orientation to getting the client's buy-in.

Validating the Client's Participation in Decision-Making

To illustrate the interaction work the psychiatrist does to validate the client's involvement in decision-making, let's consider Extract 2b (which takes place about 15 min later).

Extract 2b

```
P: We've been in: this disagreement for quite a long time.
   (1.0)
P: You're good at A:Dvocating for yourself.
   =It's good that you say what's on your mi:nd,
   and I'm going to say what I honestly think too.
   (0.6)
P: Ye know: an we're just in different camps on this one.
   (1.2)
P: I wish I could be: (0.2)
C: W'ahm recordin every meetin from now o:n.
   (0.5)
C: I'm (0.4) b-bringin my tape recorder'n: (.) recordin
   every meetin,
   (0.6)
C: Cuz y'all ain't gonna get me.
   (0.6)
C: Like y'all get me la:st ti:me.
   (1.0)
P: Well we're not- (.) Whadda ye mean get you.
   (0.4)
C: Raise my meds (or some bull[shit)
P:                            [Aw:: (.) Yeah ye-I
   ↑don't think↑ anybody's seen any:thing that makes
   us think #at this point you need your meds raised,#
   #So (0.7) #uh: <But you're: (0.2) ye know you can
   certainly do what you wan' in terms of recor:ding,
   (0.6)
P: uhm: (1.2) But WE godda do: (0.6) I godda do: as
   a prescriber what I think (0.4) is the right thing
   (0.9) from what I see and know.
   (0.8)
P: And I know I'm not inside you so I can't see it in the
   same wa:y, (0.2) but I have to go on what I see from
   the ou:tside, (0.8) and what (0.2) I know from (0.2)
   the years I've been doin this.=An it- To me it looked
   like you needed more medication. And NOW it looks like
   this amount's workin pretty good.
```

First observe that, in lines 44–46, the psychiatrist compliments the client for being a good advocate for himself. In this way, the psychiatrist validates the client's right to be an active participant in making decisions about his care. In line 48, the psychiatrist formulates them as being *in different camps*, which presents the client and the psychiatrist as having an equal standing in this debate. Later, after getting sidetracked by the client's (apparent) threat to record future meetings (lines 51–67), the psychiatrist returns to the treatment decision. In lines 69–70, she draws on her institutional identity *as a prescriber* to account for her overruling of the client's wishes. In other words, she presents herself as having the professional responsibility and the legal authority to make the decision, even if it goes against the client's wishes (Angell & Bolden, 2015). (Note that in this particular setting, the prescribed treatment is compulsory.) In lines 71–76, the psychiatrist continues to account for this decision as the *right* one for the client by prefacing her refusal to concede to the client's demand with an explicit formulation of her epistemic authority, grounding this authority in what she *sees from the outside* and what she knows from her *years* of experience (Angell & Bolden, 2015).

Overall, this segment shows that, even while making a unilateral decision in the face of the client's active resistance, the psychiatrist orients to the client's involvement in the decision-making process as valid and her decision as in need of justification.

Discussion

In this chapter, we have examined some of the ways in which psychiatrists and their clients navigate psychiatric treatment decisions. Focusing on the psychiatrist's uptake of clients' requests for medication changes, we have shown that the psychiatrist works to validate and encourage client's involvement in treatment decisions. The analysis has identified several interactional practices through which this is accomplished. First, the psychiatrist may launch interrogative series to assess grounds for the clients' request; by taking the request seriously, the psychiatrist validates clients' rights to produce the request in the first place. Second, the psychiatrist may agree with clients' diagnostic assessments (on which a medication change request may be based) and compliment them on their observations, thereby treating clients as accurate observers and reporters of their health status. Third, the psychiatrist may articulate treatment plans as collaborative (using the collective *we*) and pursue clients' acceptance of the treatment decision, thereby making clients active participants in their treatment. Finally, even when no agreement about the treatment can be reached, the psychiatrist may compliment clients for their advocacy so as to validate and encourage their active participation in decision-making.

Overall, the chapter furthers our understanding of patient advocacy in psychiatry and across medical contexts (Angell & Bolden, 2015, 2016; Bolden & Angell, 2017; Bolden et al., 2019; Gill, 2005; Gill, Halkowski, & Roberts, 2001; Kushida & Yamakawa, 2015; McCabe et al., 2013; Quirk, Chaplin, Lelliott, & Seale, 2012; Robinson, 2001; Stivers, 2002, 2007). The findings presented here have important implications for advancing our understanding of shared decision-making in psychiatry. Previous research suggests that patients may hesitate to assert themselves in clinical encounters out of deference to clinician authority (Frosch, May, Rendle, Tietbohl, & Elwyn, 2012; Woltmann & Whitley, 2010). It is, therefore, valuable to explore interactional practices through which mental health practitioners validate and encourage patients' participation in treatment decision-making.

Acknowledgements This study was funded by the Center on Adherence and Self-Determination (CASD; NIMH P20MH085981). We also acknowledge particularly the efforts of Colleen Mahoney in study design and data collection.

References

Allness, D. J., & Knoedler, W. H. (2003). *A manual for ACT start-up: Based on the PACT model of community treatment for persons with severe and persistent mental illnesses*. Arlington, VA: National Alliance for the Mentally Ill.

Angell, B., & Bolden, G. B. (2015). Justifying medication decisions in mental health care: Psychiatrists' accounts for treatment recommendations. *Social Science and Medicine, 138,* 44–56.

Angell, B., & Bolden, G. B. (2016). Team work in action: Building grounds for psychiatric medication decisions in assertive community treatment. In M. O'Reilly & J. Lester (Eds.), *Handbook of adult mental health: Discourse and conversation studies* (pp. 371–393). London: Palgrave Macmillan.

Angell, B., Matthews, E., Stanhope, V., & Rowe, M. (2015). Shared decision making. In P. Corrigan (Ed.), *Person-centered care for mental illness: The evolution of adherence and self-determination for people with mental illness*. Washington, DC: American Psychological Association.

Bolden, G. B. (2009). Implementing incipient actions: The discourse marker "so" in English conversation. *Journal of Pragmatics, 41*(5), 974–998.

Bolden, G. B., & Angell, B. (2017). The organization of the treatment recommendation phase in routine psychiatric visits. *Research on Language & Social Interaction, 50*(2), 151–170.

Bolden, G. B., Angell, B., & Hepburn, A. (2019). How clients solicit medication changes in psychiatry. *Sociology of Health & Illness, 41*(2), 411–426.

Boyd, E., & Heritage, J. (2006). Taking the history: Questioning during comprehensive history-taking. In J. Heritage & D. W. Maynard (Eds.), *Communication in medical care: Interactions between primary care physicians and patients* (pp. 151–184). Cambridge: Cambridge University Press.

Carter, M. (2003). The relationship of a self-reported assessment of need in mental illness to insight. *Journal of Mental Health, 12*(1), 81–89.

Corrigan, P., Angell, B., Davidson, L., Marcus, S. C., Salzer, M. S., Kottsieper, P., … Stanhope, V. (2012). From adherence to self-determination: Evolution of a treatment paradigm for people with serious mental illnesses. *Psychiatric Services, 63*(2), 169–173.

Curl, T. S., & Drew, P. (2008). Contingency and action: A comparison of two forms of requesting. *Research on Language and Social Interaction, 41*(2), 129–153.

Drake, R., & Deegan, P. (2009). Shared decision making is an ethical imperative. *Psychiatric Services, 60*(8), 1007.

Frosch, D. L., May, S. G., Rendle, K. A., Tietbohl, C., & Elwyn, G. (2012). Authoritarian physicians and patients' fear of being labeled "difficult" among key obstacles to shared decision making. *Health Affairs, 31*(5), 1030–1038.

Gill, V. T. (2005). Patient "demand" for medical interventions: Exerting pressure for an offer in a primary care clinic visit. *Research on Language and Social Interaction, 38*(4), 451–479.

Gill, V. T., Halkowski, T., & Roberts, C. (2001). Accomplishing a request without making one: A single case analysis of a primary care visit. *Text, 21*(1/2), 55–81.

Hepburn, A., & Bolden, G. B. (2017). *Transcribing for social research.* London: Sage.

Hepburn, A., & Potter, J. (2011). Threats: Power, family mealtimes and social influence. *British Journal of Psychology, 50*(1), 99–120.

Heritage, J. (1998). *Oh*-prefaced responses to inquiry. *Language in Society, 27*(3), 291–334.

Heritage, J. (2013). Epistemics in conversation. In J. Sidnell & T. Stivers (Eds.), *Handbook of conversation analysis* (pp. 370–394). Boston: Wiley-Blackwell.

Heritage, J., & Raymond, G. (2005). The terms of agreement: Indexing epistemic authority and subordination in talk-in-interaction. *Social Psychology Quarterly, 68*(1), 15–38.

Heritage, J., & Watson, D. R. (1979). Formulations as conversational objects. In G. Psathas (Ed.), *Everyday language: Studies in ethnomethodology* (pp. 123–162). New York: Irvington.

Kitzinger, C., & Mandelbaum, J. S. (2013). Word selection and social identities in talk. *Communication Monographs, 80*(2), 176–198.

Koenig, C. J., Wingard, L. M., Sabee, C., Olsher, D., & Vandergriff, I. (2014). Managing patient-centered communication across the type 2 diabetes illness trajectory: A grounded practical theory of interactional sensitivity. *Journal of Applied Communication Research, 42*(3), 244–267.

Kushida, S., Hiramoto, T., & Yamakawa, Y. (2016). Patients' practices for taking the initiative in decision-making in outpatient psychiatric consultations. *Communication & Medicine, 13*(2), 169–184.

Kushida, S., & Yamakawa, Y. (2015). Fitting proposals to their sequential environment: A comparison of turn designs for proposing treatment in ongoing outpatient psychiatric consultations in Japan. *Sociology of Health & Illness, 37*(4), 522–544.

Land, V., Parry, R., & Seymour, J. (2017). Communication practices that encourage and constrain shared decision making in health-care encounters: Systematic review of conversation analytic research. *Health Expectations, 20*(6), 1228–1247.

McCabe, R., Healey, P. G., Priebe, S., Lavelle, M., Dodwell, D., Laugharne, R., ... Bremner, S. (2013). Shared understanding in psychiatrist-patient communication: Association with treatment adherence in schizophrenia. *Patient Education and Counseling, 93*(1), 73–79.

Olfson, M., Marcus, S. C., Wilk, J., & West, J. C. (2006). Awareness of illness and nonadherence to antipsychotic medications among persons with schizophrenia. *Psychiatric Services, 57*(2), 205–211.

Peräkylä, A. (1998). Authority and accountability: The delivery of diagnosis in primary health care. *Social Psychology Quarterly, 61*(4), 301–320.

Quirk, A., Chaplin, R., Lelliott, P., & Seale, C. (2012). How pressure is applied in shared decisions about antipsychotic medication: A conversation analytic study of psychiatric outpatient consultations. *Sociology of Health & Illness, 34*(1), 95–113.

Raymond, C. W. (2017). Indexing a contrast: The "do"-construction in English conversation. *Journal of Pragmatics, 118*, 22–37.
Robinson, J. D. (2001). Asymmetry in action: Sequential resources in the negotiation of a prescription request. *Text, 21*(1/2), 19–54.
Robinson, J. D. (2003). An interactional structure of medical activities during acute visits and its implications for patients' consultations. *Health Communication, 25*(1), 97–123.
Robinson, J. D. (2006). Soliciting patients' presenting concerns. In J. Heritage & D. W. Maynard (Eds.), *Communication in medical care: Interaction between primary care physicians and patients* (pp. 22–47). Cambridge: Cambridge University Press.
Sacks, H., Schegloff, E. A., & Jefferson, G. (1974). A simplest systematics for the organization of turn-taking for conversation. *Language, 50*(4), 696–735.
Schegloff, E. A. (1982). Discourse as an interactional achievement: some uses of 'uh huh' and other things that come between sentences. In D. Tannen (Ed.), *Analyzing discourse: Text and talk* (pp. 71–93). Washington, DC: Georgetown University Press.
Schegloff, E. A. (2007). *Sequence organization in interaction: A primer in conversation analysis*. Cambridge: Cambridge University Press.
Sidnell, J., & Stivers, T. (Eds.). (2013). *The handbook of conversation analysis*. Oxford: Blackwell.
Stivers, T. (2002). Participating in decisions about treatment: Overt parent pressure for antibiotic medication in pediatric encounters. *Social Science and Medicine, 54*(7), 1111–1130.
Stivers, T. (2005). Modified repeats: One method for asserting primary rights from second position. *Research on Language and Social Interaction, 38*(2), 131–158.
Stivers, T. (2007). *Prescribing under pressure: Parent-physician conversations and antibiotics*. New York: Oxford University Press.
Thompson, L., & McCabe, R. (2017). How psychiatrists recommend treatment and its relationship with patient uptake. *Health Communication, 33*(11), 1345–1354.
Woltmann, E. M., & Whitley, R. (2010). Shared decision making in public mental health care: Perspectives from consumers living with severe mental illness. *Psychiatric Rehabilitation Journal, 34*(1), 29–36.
Zimmerman, D. H. (1984). Talk and its occasion: The case of calling the police. In D. Schiffrin (Ed.), *Meaning, form and use in context: Linguistic applications* (pp. 210–228). Washington, DC: Georgetown University Press.

8

Writing: A Versatile Resource in the Treatment of the Clients' Proposals

Camilla Lindholm, Melisa Stevanovic, Taina Valkeapää, and Elina Weiste

Writing in Face-to-Face Social Interaction

Research of writing has a long history. However, this research has typically focused on the dichotomy between spoken and written language, stressing the differences between situated processes of speaking

C. Lindholm (✉)
Faculty of Information Technology and Communication Sciences, Tampere University, Tampere, Finland
e-mail: camilla.lindholm@tuni.fi

M. Stevanovic
Social Sciences, University of Helsinki, Helsinki, Finland
e-mail: melisa.stevanovic@helsinki.fi

T. Valkeapää
University of Helsinki, Helsinki, Finland
e-mail: taina.valkeapaa@helsinki.fi

E. Weiste
The Finnish Institute of Occupational Health, Helsinki, Finland
e-mail: elina.weiste@ttl.fi

C. Lindholm et al. (eds.), *Joint Decision Making in Mental Health*,
The Language of Mental Health, https://doi.org/10.1007/978-3-030-43531-8_8

and of written texts. Thus, spoken language has been studied from a process perspective, while research into written language has focused on the final product.

The study of writing as a dynamic activity has been non-linear, emerging as unrelated approaches in fields like literature, socio-ethnography, and psycholinguistics. In these research domains, texts have not been studied as fixed objects but rather as possible versions among many, as embedded in the wider complex of human contextualized activities, and as cognitive processes of writing documented by technological tools. In the emerging conversation analytic research field of writing-in-interaction (Komter, 2006; Mondada & Svinhufvud, 2016), the research on writing as a process has been developed further by involving interactional and embodied aspects in the analysis. In this development, writing has been studied not only as a cognitive process but also as a social practice.

Previous research on institutional interaction has mostly focused on differences between discussions in spoken language and the written texts resulting from these discussions. In an early study of police interrogations, Jönsson and Linell (1991) demonstrated several differences between the narrative structure of the spoken interviews and the written documents. For example, the transformation from interview to document involves a higher degree of precision, increased coherence, and modification of emotionality into objectively identified findings. Similar results were demonstrated in Van Charldorp's (2014) more recent study on police interrogations. Komter (2006) further showed the interactive process that transforms a police interrogation into a written document, explaining how the coordination of participants' speaking with typing generates a monologue-like written document presenting the suspect's statement.

As summarized by Mondada and Svinhufvud (2016), previous research has outlined a few sequential environments where writing occupies a specific sequential slot. Writing has especially been studied as a closing third action following an adjacency pair. For example, the above-mentioned study on police interrogations by Komter (2006), as well as Pälli and Lehtinen's (2014) account of appraisal interviews, deal with writing as a third action in this context.

Another context investigated by many researchers is writing as a third action after a proposal and an acceptance. For example, writing as part of proposal sequences has been studied by Asmuss and Oshima (2012), Pälli and Lehtinen (2014), Nissi (2015), and Mondada and Svinhufvud (2016). In their study of appraisal interviews, Pälli and Lehtinen (2014) showed that moving into writing usually demonstrates unproblematic acceptance of a proposal, whereas a delay indicates that the decision is somewhat problematic and is a matter of negotiation.

Writing also relates to the processes of decision-making in institutional interaction. In analyzing instances of note-taking in decision-making, Stevanovic (2013) illuminated how writing may be a manner of individually registering a final decision. Nissi (2015) demonstrated how shared text production in multiparty meetings involves two forms of decision-making. First, the group must make decisions about local text production that involve what to write in the text. Second, a more general decision is involved, because the written document will commit the group members to carrying out certain public service in the future. Thus, by agreeing with the local formulations of the document, the meeting participants also agree to provide future services.

Once formulated, texts become independent entities in organizational life, and new organization members no longer have access to the processes preceding the formulation of the documents (Nissi, 2015; cf. Pälli, Vaara, & Sorsa, 2009 on strategy documents). As demonstrated by Moore, Whalen, and Gathman (2010), documents can coordinate organizational activity and play a constitutional role in the entire activity systems of organizations. Drawing on the relationship between texts and organizational constitution, Cooren (2004, 2009) introduced the notion of textual agency, stating that texts themselves, not just the people producing and using the texts, make a difference in organizations by performing various actions. Cooren (2004, 2009) adapted the notion of the speech act (Austin, 1975; Searle, 1989) to written text, postulating the ability of texts to perform certain speech acts. Originally, Austin (1975) introduced two types of speech acts: constatives are statements that can be either true or false (e.g., "The sun is shining today"), and performatives are statements that produce actions (e.g., "I sentence you to prison"). Although speech acts were originally considered to be instances of face-to-face spoken communication, legal documents have been studied as written indications of speech acts (Fiorito, 2006; Visconti, 2009).

Written documents of the type analyzed in the present study are not performative in the sense of legal language, which creates "deontic states that are made obligatory by law" (Fiorito, 2006, p. 103). However, these documents can still be considered as performatives from the whole organization's perspective. As demonstrated (e.g., Nissi, 2015), written documentation turns ideas into guidelines that play a fundamental role in the organization. In this chapter, writing is analyzed as a resource for decision-making in the mental rehabilitation context of the Clubhouse organization (described in more detail in Chapters 2, 6, 9, and 12). The following conversational extract provides a first glimpse into how strongly writing is associated with decision-making in the everyday activities of the Clubhouse. Here, Clubhouse member Ada acts as secretary, writing with a keyboard, while the text-in-production was projected on the wall.

Extract 1

```
01 SW1: mutta me ei ehkä voida sitä tähän ainakaan vielä
        but maybe we can't put it here at least not yet

02      laittaa koska me ei olla tehty sitä päätöstä se
        because we haven't made that decision it

03      on vasta huomenna nyt sitte se meijän
        is not until tomorrow now then the wrapping up

04      kehittämispäivän purku
        of our development day

05      (1.0)

06 SW1: ni onks se vähän (0.2) sit me ei ehkä voida
        so is it a bit (0.2) then we can't perhaps

07      sitä tohon vielä laittaa (.) sit me ollaan ikään
        put it there yet (.) then we have kind of

08      kuin se jo päätetty että se täytyy ottaa tähän
        already decided it that we need to include it

09      osaksi,
        here

10 Ada: mmh

11 SW1: vaik se päätetään vasta huomenna.
        even if we make the decision tomorrow

12 Ada: nii.
        yes

13      (2.0)

14 SW1: joo (.) me voidaan se sit lisätä nää voi
        yes (.) we can then add it these can
```

15 kuitenkin kun nää tallennetaan tänne nii tota
still when we save these here then erm

16 ne voidaan sitte muokkailla
we can then edit them

17 sitä mukaan kun (0.2) mutta millä me saadaan toi
at the same time as (0.2) but how do we get that

18 jos me tulostetaan toi eka dia?
one if we print the first slide

In Extract 1, the support worker SW1 repeatedly expresses the connection between writing something down and making a decision. As seen in line 1, she begins by pointing out that the group cannot write down a point about making individual rehabilitation/career plans for the Clubhouse members. As an explanation, she mentions (lines 2–4) that the decision has not been made yet but will be made the following day. After a pause, she repeats (lines 6–8) that they cannot write something down yet: "Then we can't perhaps put it there yet." She continues to mention that writing something down signals making a decision ("Then we have kind of already decided it," lines 7–8).

Clubhouse member Ada acknowledges SW1's statement by producing minimal response tokens (lines 10, 12), after which SW1 states that the information can be added and the texts edited later. In this, SW1 implies that the text can be completed once the decision has been made. At this point, SW1 initiates talk about practical issues related to ongoing tasks—how pieces of cardboard should be placed on the wall (line 17 onwards). Once she has indicated that new information can be added to the text later, she moves on to discussing other matters.

Extract 1 illustrates how closely connected collective writing was to decision-making in group meetings at the Clubhouse, as made explicit by the support worker. This connection makes writing a fruitful domain for study in the field of joint decision-making. Therefore, this article focuses on three different uses of writing in various stages of decision-making:

1. Initial stage: How are ideas transformed into proposals during the initial stages of decision-making?
2. Mid-stage: How does editing texts contribute to decision-making?
3. Final stage: What is the status of written texts? Are they considered to be tentative proposals or finalized decisions?

Data and Method

The data analyzed for this chapter were collected as part of a larger project on mental health rehabilitation (see Chapter 2 for a description of the project). Recorded over an 11-month period at a Finnish Clubhouse, the 29 hours of video data featured authentic interactions from group meetings involving 2–10 clients and 1–3 support workers. The data collection was based on participants' informed consent, and research permission was obtained from the Clubhouse organization board in the relevant area.

The group investigated in this study was a work coaching group open to Clubhouse members. The group discussed a range of topics, from future employment plans to generic skills needed in the labor market. The generic skills practiced during the sessions involved active participation at the meetings.

Examining the data with the overall aim of studying the decision-making processes revealed that the Clubhouse meetings were characterized by the support workers' attempts to promote clients' participation. Furthermore, texts and joint writing played an important role in the interaction. At the beginning of every meeting, a client was chosen to be a secretary in charge of taking minutes. Besides the minutes, other texts like guidelines for Clubhouse activities were also written and edited during the meetings. These texts were often written on a computer and reflected onto a screen.

In this study, the focus was on how the writing processes related to decision-making, and it identified the role of writing in various stages of decision-making. This role is the focus of analysis in this chapter. In section "Analysis: Three Uses of Writing During Joint Decision-Making

Processes", the results of the analysis are presented. Because the authors did not have access to all texts written during the meetings, this analysis concentrates on writing as a process rather than the written products.

Conversation analysis was the method used (cf. Chapter 1 for an introduction of conversation analysis and the study of joint decision-making). This chapter draws on the conversation analytic literature introduced above.

Analysis: Three Uses of Writing During Joint Decision-Making Processes

In this section, we discuss how writing relates to decision-making in the data. In their account of writing-in-interaction, Mondada and Svinhufvud (2016) distinguished between moving into writing and actual writing; they then analyzed both phenomena as embodied conduct. The present study does not distinguish between different phases in the writing process. Instead, this presentation of cases follows the phases of the decision-making process, proceeding from the initial phase to the final phase of decision-making via the mid-stage.

Transforming Tentative Ideas into Proposals

During the initial stage of a decision-making process, writing allows even tentative ideas expressed by Clubhouse members to be transformed into proposals with potential future consequences. This is the case for Extract 2. Here, the group is discussing upcoming meetings.

Extract 2

01 Ari: kyllä sitä oppii t- tekemällä (-)
you do learn by doing

02 SW1: mm

03 SW2: mm

04 SW1: kun tässä tulee nyt kuitenkin ihan (.) siis hyviä
when we now have really (.) good

05 ideoita mitä me voitas tehdä tässä et pitäskö
ideas what we could do so should we

06 SW2: mm

07 SW1: niitä laittaa ↑ylös paperille et muuten me ei
write them down on paper because otherwise we

08 [muisteta näitä.] haluaaks joku. (0.5)
won't remember them does anybody want to (0.5)

09 SW2: [laitetaan]
let's put them down

10 haluaksä Kai pistää
do you Kai want to put

11 SW1: sä oot hyvä (.) kirjuri (-)((naurua))
you're a good (.) secretary (-) ((laughter))

12 Kai: no no ku mää (.) lähen jo (.) joudun lähtee
well well when I (.) already go (.) have to go

13 ↑kymmenen minuutin sisällä kun mul on se, (1.0)
in 10 minutes when I have that, (1.0)

14 (muuten voisin kirjoittaa) (--)
(otherwise I could write) (--)

15 SW1: voiksää Asko laittaa paperille
can you Asko write down

```
16          (.)

17  SW1:  et
          you can't

18  SW1:  (kuka on täs)
          (who is here)

19  Mia:  (--)

20  SW1:  Ari voi ottaa
          Ari can take

21        (.)

22  Ari:  (-) minä otan tämän sihteerin homman
          (-) I take this  secretary work

23  SW1:  no ni,
          okay,

24        (.)

25  SW1:  niin mä aattelin et tässähän tuli yks, (0.8)
          so I thought that we had one,(0.8)

26        [yks idea
          one idea

27  SW2:  [mm joo
           mm yes

28 SW1:   Kailla (.) (--) laittaa vähän ranskiksia sinne
          from Kai (.) (--) write down some bullet points

29        (-) ylös voidaan sit miettiä,
          (-) we can discuss them then

30  Ari:  mikä se [oli.
          what was it

31  SW1:          [elikkä, (1.2) sulla oli vähän ninku
                  so (1.2) you had a bit like

32        sitä (.) <oman toiminnan arviointia>
          that (.) assessment of one's own activity
```

In Extract 2, one member has presented the idea of going to the employment office to learn something new, and this has sparked a discussion. In line 4, the support worker SW1 (a) defines a member's prior, rather unspecified, turns as suggestions for further activities ("really good ideas what we could do," lines 4–5), (b) suggests writing these ideas down ("should we write them down on paper," lines 5–7), and (c) addresses one of the members as the potential secretary ("do you Kai want to put," line 10). Her turn is followed by a negotiation about who should act as secretary (lines 8–19). After the negotiation, SW1 returns to the matter of writing things down. She refers to an idea introduced by another member ("one idea from Kai," lines 25, 28) and the importance of writing this idea down ("write down some bullet points," lines 28–29). After the member acting as secretary asks for help formulating the ideas, SW1 reformulates Kai's idea (lines 31–32).

As seen in this extract, SW1 referred to the ideas presented by various Clubhouse members and proposed the importance of writing these ideas down. She even explicitly pointed to the opportunity to discuss the proposals later (line 29). Thus, vague ideas achieved the status of proposals through the process of writing them down. Simultaneously, the process of writing down ideas did not necessarily entail commitment to accepting the proposal. Instead, the written-down text embodied the possibility that the proposal might be returned to and accepted later. This allowed the participants to display their "in principle" serious engagement with the proposal, even if they moved on to a new topic.

Extract 3 provides another example of how unspecific ideas are transformed into proposals by formulating these ideas in text.

Extract 3

```
01  Ira: ja vähän harjotella sitä et miten se lähtee.
         and practice a bit how it goes

02  SW2: mm,

03  SW1: ↑voidaanhan käydä esimerkiks joku kerta
         we can for example at some point have a (.)

04       sellanen (.) keskustelu että että tota (.)
         discussion that erm (.)

05       vaikka sillon jos tulee näitäkin (.) jäseniä
         for example if there are members coming

06       jotka on, (0.3) sieltä Helsingistä jotka on,
         who are, (0.3) from Helsinki who have

07       (0.3) on tota noin niin käyny [sen, ]
         (0.3) have erm well erm gone through that

08 SW2:                               [mm-m,] mm-m,

09 SW1: tehny siirtymätyöjaksoja (.) ja sitten meillä
        done transition work periods (.) and then we

10      on henkilökuntajäseninä,(0.4) kokemusta siitä
        have as staff members (0.4) experience of how

11      että miten se prosessi niinku menee kun se työ
        the process goes when one starts the work

12      alotetaan et jos mennään sitte jo siihen
        so if we already go to that

13      pisteeseen, (0.3) ja mietitään
        point (0.3) and think about

14      sitä niin voidaan käydä ihan hyvin (.)
        that then nothing prevents us from having (.)

15      semmon[enki] keskustelu, (0.4) [jollaki kertaa]
        that kind of conversation (0.4) at some point

16 SW2:       [mm, ]                   [se ois hyvä   ]
               mm                      that would be good
```

```
17  SW1: et mitä siinä että mitä siinä ↑tapahtuu ihan
         that what happens there

18       konkreettisesti että, (0.4) miten se työ yhdessä
         concretely that (0.4) what the work we

19       harjotellaan ja, (0.4) palkkaussysteemit ja
         practice together and (0.4) salary systems and so

20       muut. ↑Pitäskö seki laittaa sinne ylös.
         forth. Should we also write that down

         ((lines omitted))

21  Aki: mikä se työalotusprosessi (.) mitä sinne piti
         what the process of starting work (.) what should

22       kirjottaa
         I write

23  SW2: oisko se työnaloitusprosessi ja
         should we write the process of starting work and

24       työvalmentajan tuki. ehkä me siitä
         the support from the work coach. maybe we'll

25       muistetaan mitä se
         remember what it
```

Extract (3) features a lengthy discussion about a potential future activity—arranging an event at which the process of transition work will be discussed. In line 3, SW1 expresses herself vaguely by saying that they can arrange a discussion "at some point." However, she then describes the future event in detail by outlining several aspects worth discussing at the event (lines 17–20). In line 20, she suggests that this idea be written down. The member acting as secretary asks about how he should formulate the idea when writing it down (line 21). In this case, the member identifies the "process of starting work" as the core of the support worker's proposal and then asks the support workers for clarification about the linguistic formulation of the proposal. SW2 responds by providing a formulation and then referring to the fact that they may need to remember the idea later: ("maybe we'll remember," lines 24–25). The process of collective writing becomes visible in how the parties negotiate the precise formulations in lines 22–23.

Hence, the proposal was discussed and dealt with in the interaction, but more detailed planning was postponed. The suggestion was considered; it was written down, and the need to remember it in the future was referenced. However, no decision was made. Writing the suggestion down paused the discussion. Both Extracts 2 and 3 exemplify how tentative ideas were taken seriously and treated as proposals that must be considered.

Text Editing as a Path to Proposal Content

Writing may also constitute the "core" of the participants' negotiations about the content of the decisions to be made. In this case, texts written on other occasions are used as a starting point for decision-making, which is realized by the participants' joint text editing. In other words, editing texts prompts several decisions concerning both the content and linguistic formulations of the text.

In their prompts to launch editing activities, the support workers frequently followed a dual agenda, on one hand, asking about the clients' grasp of the meaning of the text and, on the other hand, about the acceptability of a given linguistic formulation. This agenda allowed members to contribute freely to the unfolding interaction while also allowing the support workers to monitor the Clubhouse members' epistemic access to the proposal content, intervening when needed. These processes are exemplified in Extracts 4 and 5.

In Extract 4, a text produced in another context is made visible on the screen, and the support worker is typing on the computer while simultaneously using the text as a basis for discussion. In line 1, she points at the screen and asks the group about their opinion of the text. Her question has an open format ("what do you think"), which does not restrict the requested responses in any way. In line 5, however, she produces a more specific two-part question, in which she asks for the group's opinion about both the form ("is this ok") and the content ("what does this mean") of the featured text. The response from the group is minimal; only one member responds minimally (line 7), and a lengthy pause (line 8) follows. Then, SW1 poses a new question to the group (line 9).

Extract 4

```
01 SW1: no tää seuraava, (.) mitä ootte mieltä.
        so this next one (.) what do you think

       ((points at a point visible on the screen)

02     (5.0) ((the group looks at the screen))

03 SW1: mä vaihdan tän näin.
        I'll change this one like this.

04      (10.0)

05 SW1: onks tää ookoo ja mitä tää tarkottaa.
        is this ok and what does this mean

06     (1.0)

07 Ira: on.
        yes

08      (4.0)

09 SW1: voidaaks me kirjata tätä tähän koska siis
        can we write this down here because

10      tää on nyt, (.) otettu mallia toisista
        this is now (.) we took the model from other

11      klubitaloista sielähä on tämmönen, (.) ura
        clubhouses they use this kind of (.) career

12      kautta kuntoutussuunnitelma. (.) ja meillä on,
        slash rehabilitation plan (.) and we have

13      (0.8) ollu toisella nimellä. (0.8)
        (0.8) used another name (0.8)
```

```
14          tavotesuunnitelma. (0.4) (mitä näitä)
            target plan (0.4) (what there)

15          (.)

16 Ira:     must toi on i[ha
            I think that's quite

17 SW1:                  [et se on pitäny [olla siinä
                         that it needed to be there

18 Ira:                                   [sellane lyhyt ja
                                           a short and

19          ytimekäs toi ehdotus.
            succinct that suggestion

20          (0.8)

21 SW1:     mutta meil ei välttämättä
            but at our place we don't necessarily

22          tarvii, (.) tehdä sitä. (1.4) suunnitelmaa.
            need to (.) do that (1.4) plan

23          (2.0)

24 Ira:     no pitäskö sinne laittaa että haluttaessa.
            well should we write down that when desired
```

The support worker's turn (line 9) contains an initial question, ("can we write this down here"), followed by a causal clause initiated with the subordinating conjunction *koska* ("because"). The causal clause provides a background to the question; SW1 points out that they have used a text produced at another Clubhouse as a model for the text on which they are currently working. Furthermore, she outlines the differences between the terms various Clubhouses use to refer to certain documents utilized in their everyday activities. One of the Clubhouse members, Ira, agrees with SW1's suggestion (line 16). However, Ira interrupts her turn, because SW1 overlaps by referring to a certain point that must be expressed if the group wants to follow the other Clubhouse's model verbatim (line 17). Ira then completes her turn (lines 18–19), expressing acceptance of SW1's initial suggestion. In line 21, however, SW1 adds a contrasting remark, *mutta* ("but"), stating that they do not necessarily need to follow this model. Thus, she expresses the group's freedom to take an independent position toward the text they use as a basis for their negotiations. Ira suggests (line 24) a reformulation of the already-written text, indicating how they can change the text to be more flexible and not overly dependent on the other Clubhouse's model.

In Extract 4, the negotiations were related to editing a previously written text to meet the needs of the current group. The support worker asked questions both about the form and content of the text in creation, thus treating the Clubhouse members as peers who had a say in how the text was formulated. In this instance, text editing was a collective process.

Extract 5 features an example of a negotiation which involves two support workers and a Clubhouse member as participants.

Extract 5

```
01 SW3: must tääl on aika kivasti tää et
        I think this is quite nicely put this that

02      siirtymätyö on jäsenoikeus ei
        transition work is the right of a member not an

03      velvote(.) vähän liittyy tähän et ei jos
        obligation (.) this has a little to do with this

04      ei niiku, (.) ei kenenkään oo pakko lähtee.
        that if you don't (.) nobody has to go
        ((reads from a paper))

05 Tia: nii toiki on ihan hyvä pointti.
        yes that's a good point too

06 SW1: no laitetaan seki tohon.
        ok let's put it there then
```

The sequence begins with SW3 evaluating a formulation in an already-written text. First, she frames the formulation in a positive way. Second, she reads aloud from the text, "Transition work is the right of a member, not an obligation." Finally, she reformulates the cited text in her own words, defining the message of the text as follows: nobody has to attend transition work against their will. Tia gives positive feedback (line 5), and her turn is followed by SW1's turn, in which SW1 immediately agrees to write down the formulation. Thus, they choose to accept the formulation as such, without any changes or further negotiations. Unlike Extract 4, no lengthy negotiation about using the already-written text as material for the text-in-production can be found in this extract.

Extracts 4 and 5 illustrated how text editing forms the basis for negotiations between clients and support workers, providing the clients with an opportunity to contribute to both the content and linguistic formulations of the texts they are editing.

Ambiguous Status of the Already-Written Texts

During the final stages of the decision-making process, the text the group has been working on can be a resource when trying to reach a decision after lengthy negotiations. However, the status of already-written texts as tentative proposals versus confirmed decisions is ambiguous and negotiable. Therefore, this section demonstrates these negotiations' delicate balance between the ideals of consensus-based decision-making and more pragmatic considerations about the group's needs. Extract 6 (analyzed at length in Chapter 12) features the end of a long discussion about the coaching group's name. Here, writing is done with a pen, not on the computer.

Extract 6

```
01 Leo: miksi me päätimme tämän.
        what have we decided

02 Anu: laita se työvalmennus.
        write down the work coaching

03 SW1: käyks se (.) käyks se kaikille.
        is it (.) is it okay for everybody

04 Esa: eiks melkein kaikki sitä äänestäny.
        didn't almost everyone vote for that option

05 SW1: no Maj ehdotti kyl toista ja mä: mulle kävi
        well Maj suggested something else and I'm okay

06      kaikki, (.) kaikki k(h)äy,
        with everything

07      (2.0)

08 Anu: niin no se on nyt sittee se.
        so well that's now what it is

09      (1.0)

10 Anu: päätös tapahtu (--) demokratia (-) vai
        the decision was made (--) democracy (-) or

11      (3.0)

12 Ida:  sillä nyt melkeen
         because now almost

13 Anu: ja kun se on vielä kuulakärkikynä niin sitä
        and when it's a ball pen then it

14      ei enää voi pyyhkii.
        can't be erased anymore

15      (0.5)

16 Maj: voi sen sotkee ja kirjottaa uuden.
        well one can mess it up and write again
```

In line 1, Leo again asks what name they should choose. Anu (line 2) encourages him to write down this choice, and Esa (line 4) supports the decision by stating that almost everybody voted for this proposal. Anu continues, saying that it was a democratic decision, and then she says that the name was written with a ballpoint pen (lines 13–14) and thus cannot be erased. This utterance stresses the idea on which the present study is based; at the Clubhouse, writing and decision-making are intimately connected. Because the name suggestion has been written down, it cannot be erased; thus, the decision has been made through writing down the name. Although nobody has declared that a decision has been made (cf. Austin, 1975), Anu retrospectively treats the act of writing down a name as a decision that could not be altered.

However, Maj, who makes another suggestion, declares her divergent opinion (line 16); she points out that the text can be messed up and rewritten. This conversation can be interpreted as a discussion about textual agency (Cooren, 2004, 2009) in which Anu treats the written text as having independent agency, whereas Maj ascribes the capacity to make decisions to the present human actors. According to Maj, they have the right to change the text if they want to.

Therefore, this analysis indicates specific practical advantages of writing for managing participation and joint decision-making in mental health rehabilitation. Writing can be used to reach a decision after lengthy negotiations, enabling the conversation to move forward to other topics.

Conclusions

In this chapter, we investigated writing-in-interaction at the Clubhouse. Writing has been studied as a joint and collaborative practice rather than an individual and cognitive phenomenon. The focus has been on writing as a process, and written texts as products have been omitted from the current analysis. The present study is particularly connected to previous literature about writing on decision-making that has examined writing as typically following the actions of proposal and acceptance (Asmuss & Oshima, 2012; Mondada & Svinhufvud, 2016; Nissi, 2015;

Pälli & Lehtinen, 2014). However, as the present investigation has indicated, proposals can present as emergent processes, and identifying acceptance of proposals can be subject to negotiation. Thus, this study sheds new light on the role of writing in sequences involving proposals.

This study reported on the role of texts in various phases of the decision-making process and demonstrated how the texts achieve their own intersubjective understanding based on their connection to the various stages of decision-making. The participants oriented to the texts in different ways depending on the decision-making phase. In the initial stages, the participants oriented to the texts to transform tentative ideas into proposals; they simultaneously postponed the decision. While editing texts, various immediate decisions must be made regarding both the content and the form of the texts. During this process, the texts were used by the support workers to engage the Clubhouse members in the shared activity and allow them to provide input. Finally, texts could also conclude a lengthy negotiation, causing a decision to be made.

The present analysis has revealed that texts at the Clubhouse were developed in a manner promoting the intertextuality and intersubjectivity of the texts. Intertextuality refers to texts achieving their meaning from interconnection with other texts. In the present data, the connection between the texts-in-production and related texts became visible, especially in the processes of editing and revising texts based on those produced at other Clubhouses. The revision work launched negotiations about both the content and the form of the model texts; in other words, does the group accept this content in this form as the guidelines for their activities? The interconnectedness between the texts at the various Clubhouses revealed the structure of the Clubhouse organization, with its underlying common ideology open to renegotiation to fit the demands of the individual Clubhouse.

This analysis has demonstrated that the process of writing balanced the ideals and practice of decision-making at the Clubhouse. On one hand, decision-making at the Clubhouse promoted a consensus-based process (cf. Chapter 12) in which everybody could be involved in the decision-making. On the other hand, pragmatic decisions concerning what the group needed had to be made. As in all institutional interactions, the meetings had an agenda and an allotted time slot;

these factors constituted the outer circumstances of the interaction. Another issue related to consensus-based decision-making was the need to promote participation, which could be done by responding to Clubhouse members and involving them in collective writing.

The extracts analyzed have demonstrated how collective writing balances ideals and practice. The first section showed how the support workers encouraged writing down unspecified ideas presented by the Clubhouse members. The transformation of these ideas into text supported the delicate balance between involving Clubhouse members in the interaction and sticking to the agenda. Writing the ideas down and mentioning returning to these matters in the future gave the impression that the ideas were treated seriously and were not simply dismissed. Simultaneously, writing the ideas down enabled the conversation to move on to other matters, and the agenda was followed without requiring any decisions to be made on the proposed matters. Therefore, writing down ideas helped the support workers meet the local institutional goal of following the agenda set for the meeting while simultaneously following the overall Clubhouse ideology of involving the members in decision-making.

The Clubhouse members were involved in the collective editing of texts based on previous texts. The text editing questions the extent to which guidelines formulated in another context are applicable in the current context and whether formulations from prior texts should be accepted as such or edited and reformulated to fit the current context. The shared editing of texts enabled a discussion between support workers and Clubhouse members in which the support workers treated the members as peers and texts were formulated as a collective endeavor. During the editing process, the members were provided with the opportunity to express their opinion on both the content and linguistic formulations of the text, and this opportunity allowed the Clubhouse members to contribute to the interaction. However, the support workers acted as the party who had the final say about the text-in-production; the Clubhouse members confirmed the correct formulations to use in the text with the support workers. In this way, the support workers could both involve the Clubhouse members in interaction and monitor their access to the proposal content, ensuring that the agenda was followed.

Writing can also be a resource for concluding a lengthy decision-making process. However, the status of the written formulations as tentative proposals versus confirmed decisions is sometimes ambiguous; this status can become a topic for negotiation itself. Additionally, these negotiations were connected with balancing the Clubhouse ideal of democratic decision-making with practical considerations related to the framework of institutional talk. Sometimes, a member might stick with the agenda and move the decision-making process forward while the support worker ensured that the decision-making was consensus-based. In this instance, the support worker carried the responsibility of involving everybody in decision-making and reaching a balance between honoring the ideals of democratic decision-making and orienting to the overall conversational agenda.

References

Asmuss, B., & Oshima, S. (2012). Negotiation of entitlement in proposal sequences. *Discourse Studies, 14*(1), 67–86.

Austin, J. L. (1975). *How to do things with words*. Oxford: Oxford University Press.

Cooren, F. (2004). Textual agency: How texts do things in organizational settings. *Organization, 11*(3), 373–393.

Cooren, F. (2009). The haunting question of textual agency: Derrida and Garfinkel on iterability and eventfulness. *Research on Language and Social Interaction, 42*(1), 42–67.

Fiorito, L. (2006). On performatives in legal discourse. *Metalogicon, XIX*(2), 101–112.

Jönsson, L., & Linell, P. (1991). Story generations: From dialogical interviews to written reports in police interrogations. *Text, 11*(3), 419–440.

Komter, M. (2006). From talk to text: The interactional construction of a police record. *Research on Language and Social Interaction, 39*(3), 201–228.

Mondada, L., & Svinhufvud, K. (2016). Writing-in-interaction: Studying writing as a multimodal phenomenon in social interaction. *Language and Dialogue, 6*(1), 1–53.

Moore, R. J., Whalen, J., & Gathman, E. C. H. (2010). The work of the work order: Document practice in face-to-face service encounters. In N. Llewellyn & J. Hindmarsh (Eds.), *Organisation, interaction and practice: Studies in ethnomethodology and conversation analysis* (pp. 172–197). Cambridge: Cambridge University Press.

Nissi, R. (2015). From entry proposals to a joint statement: Practices of shared text production in multiparty meeting interaction. *Journal of Pragmatics, 79,* 1–21.

Pälli, P., & Lehtinen, E. (2014). Making objectives common in performance appraisal interviews. *Language & Communication, 39,* 92–108.

Pälli, P., Vaara, E., & Sorsa, V. (2009). Strategy as text and discursive practice: A genre-based approach to strategizing in city administration. *Discourse & Communication, 3*(3), 303–318.

Searle, J. (1989). How performatives work. *Linguistics and Philosophy, 12*(5), 535–558.

Stevanovic, M. (2013). Constructing a proposal as a thought: A way to manage problems in the initiation of joint decision-making in Finnish workplace interaction. *Pragmatics, 23,* 519–544.

Van Charldorp, T. (2014). "What happened?": From talk to text in police interrogations. *Language & Communication, 36,* 7–24.

Visconti, J. (2009). Speech acts in legal language: Introduction. *Journal of Pragmatics, 41*(3), 393–400.

9

"*What Do You Think*?" Interactional Boundary-Making Between "*You*" and "*Us*" as a Resource to Elicit Client Participation

Jenny Paananen, Camilla Lindholm, Melisa Stevanovic, Taina Valkeapää, and Elina Weiste

Communal Ideologies Related to Mental Health Rehabilitation

The title of this volume reveals the ideological concept behind decision-making in the context of mental health. The aim is to reach decisions jointly, through interaction, to involve mental health clients in the decisions that concern their treatment, services, activities, and goals (Royal College of Psychiatrists Social Inclusion Scoping Group, 2009). The Clubhouse model of psychosocial rehabilitation examined in this study is designed to promote inclusion by reducing the power

J. Paananen (✉) · M. Stevanovic · T. Valkeapää · E. Weiste
University of Helsinki, Helsinki, Finland
e-mail: jenny.paananen@helsinki.fi

M. Stevanovic
e-mail: melisa.stevanovic@helsinki.fi

T. Valkeapää
e-mail: taina.valkeapaa@helsinki.fi

C. Lindholm et al. (eds.), *Joint Decision Making in Mental Health*,
The Language of Mental Health, https://doi.org/10.1007/978-3-030-43531-8_9

differential between the rehabilitation staff and the clients, labeling the latter as members rather than clients or mental health patients (see also Chapter 2). By building on the members' abilities, the Clubhouse forms a working community, where the members and the support workers take care of all functions of the house together (Chen, 2017). All matters related to the Clubhouse activities are decided at meetings by consensus-based decision-making, which aims to consider everyone's view (Clubhouse International, 2019; Hänninen, 2012; see also Chapter 12). Instead of medical treatment, the Clubhouse uses joint activities as a path to recovery (Anthony, 2007).

In practice, however, achieving a collaborative community can be challenging and the effects of mental illnesses hard to dismiss, especially if they affect the clients' ability and willingness to participate in interaction (see e.g., Hickey & Kipping, 1998). People with long-term mental health problems can be disempowered by social isolation and may suffer from low self-image and low self-esteem (Hänninen, 2012, p. 41). It is therefore crucial that the support workers facilitate group activities and manage participation so that all clients have equal opportunities to influence the decisions.

However, the demand to manage interaction while maintaining a low hierarchy creates another controversy between ideology and practice. In a sense, the ideological concept of working as equals entails that equality is surveyed and pursued through the work of institutional agents who are in control. The institutional status and responsibilities inevitably give support workers more power than clients, and the power differential is also likely to also reflect on the interaction (see Drew & Heritage, 1992). Indeed, previous studies of Clubhouse interaction have shown that the support workers may use their position to impose

C. Lindholm
Tampere University, Tampere, Finland
e-mail: camilla.lindholm@tuni.fi

E. Weiste
Finnish Institute of Occupational Health, Helsinki, Finland
e-mail: elina.weiste@ttl.fi

decisions and to overrule clients' opinions (Karlsson, 2005; Valkeapää, Tanaka, Lindholm, Weiste, & Stevanovic, 2018).

This controversy between ideology and practice is a fruitful starting point for a conversation analytic study of the current type. In this study, our focus was on support workers' proposals. Particularly, we focused on how support workers distinguish clients from themselves by addressing them in second-person plural forms (2PL). We aim to demonstrate that these departures from *us* to *you* not only reveal the inner division between the Clubhouse clients and the staff, but also illuminate the dynamics of participation and involvement.

Selecting You to Speak Next

The principle of a conversation is that the participants take turns to talk. Ideally, only one participant at a time takes the role of the *speaker*, while the others listen, or, act as *hearers* (Goffman, 1981; Goodwin, 1981) or *recipients* (Schegloff, 1996). According to Sacks, Schegloff, and Jefferson (1974), the first rule of turn-taking is that if the current speaker selects a specific next speaker, this person should take the turn. Selecting the next speaker can be done in various ways. For example, the speaker can address a specific recipient by explicitly referring to them in the turn. Thus, the hearer becomes an *addressee* (Goodwin, 1981, cf. *ratified hearer*, Goffman, 1981). The most common way to refer to a recipient is to use a second-person reference, but recipients may also be identified with names and noun phrases (Lerner, 1996; Schegloff, 1996, on the preference of minimization in reference to persons, see Sacks & Schegloff, 1979). However, recipients can also be addressed in a non-verbal manner—for example, gazing, pointing or nodding towards a party constitutes a social signal of involvement in interaction (see e.g., Goodwin, 1981, pp. 29–30; Lerner, 1996).

In our paper, we analyze instances of support workers using second-person plural (2PL) reference forms as a resource to select the next speakers in group discussions. Interestingly, these expressions refer to multiple addressees without verbally identifying the group (*you* vs. *you clients* vs. *clients*), and therefore their reference must be interpreted through other cues on each occasion (Lerner, 1996). Unlike the 1PL reference forms that refer to a group in which the speaker is included, the 2PL references create an outgroup, a group which does not include the speaker, a group of others—and it is the others' responsibility to recognize the reference and respond to it (on ingroups and outgroups, see Tajfel, 1981). However, addressing a group of people does not necessarily oblige all of them to respond; in certain circumstances, a sole response may be enough to represent the group (Lerner, 1993).

As our data are in Finnish and our focus lies in the topic of person reference and categorization, we will now introduce three basic features of person reference in Finnish that differ from patterns of person reference in English:

1. The category of person is expressed in three coding systems: personal pronouns (*te* PRO2PL), verbal person marking (*ajattele-**tte*** think-2PL), and possessive suffixes (*teidän vuoro-**nne*** you-GEN turn-POSS "your turn") (Helasvuo & Laitinen, 2006).
2. Person is expressed both in the subject and in the predicate verb (***te*** *ajattele-**tte*** you-2PL think-2PL "you think"), but it is also possible to omit the pronominal subject and to express the person with only the verbal person marking (*ajattele-**tte*** think-2PL "you think," on subject marking, see Helasvuo & Laitinen, 2006).
3. Unlike in English, in which the pronoun *you* represents second person in both singular and plural, Finnish presents two separate pronouns: *sinä* for singular, and *te* for plural, and the verbal person marking for singular and plural differs as well (*-t* and *-tte*). The singular second-person references can also be used to create an open reference, referring to a specific experience or state of affairs on a general level (Suomalainen, 2018). However, second person in plural is not employed in this kind of use.

Research Questions

In our analysis, we proceed from the interpretation of the second-person plural references to the sequential contexts and functions of these references. Our research questions are the following:

1. Who are the referents of 2PL forms in support worker-initiated proposal sequences?
2. In what contexts do the support workers use 2PL in proposal sequences?
3. What functions does the use of 2PL serve in proposal sequences?

Data and Methods

The data consist of 29 video-recorded group discussions in a Finnish Clubhouse. The discussions (30–70 minutes) involved 2–10 clients and 1–3 support workers trained in social work. All discussions were about working life and work-related skills (see Chapter 2 for more details on the data).

A total of 450 support workers' proposals was collected and coded regarding the linguistic features. For this study, 42 proposals containing 2PL forms were selected. Hence, second-person plural is by no means a default feature in support workers' proposals, but it is not rare either.

The collection considers proposals that contain the personal pronoun *te* and/or a predicate verb that expresses second-person plural (*-tte*). There are 19 overt and 19 null second-person plural subjects in the collection. In addition, we have included four cases in which the pronoun *te* is not in a subject position but appears in an inflected form (*tulee-ks* ***te-ille*** *miel-een* come-Q you-2PL.ILL mind-ILL "does anything come to your minds"). The corresponding proposal sequences were analyzed further using multimodal conversation analysis (Sidnell & Stivers, 2013). Special attention was paid to the linguistic details, as well as to the gaze and gestures.

Second-Person Plural References in Proposal Sequences

Here, we analyze how the support workers use second-person plural references in proposal sequences. First, we ask who the support workers refer to by *you*-2PL? Second, we examine the contexts of 2PL forms and analyze the verbs and constructions 2PL relates to, and what actions *you* are expected to do. In the final two sections, we examine interactional functions that 2PL references are associated within our data: attracting attention and pursuing a response.

Who Are You?

How do we know that the second person actually refers to the clients and not to the whole group including the other present support workers? Sometimes, the exact reference is difficult to identify, but in most cases, there are cues guiding the interpretation. In this section, we demonstrate some of the linguistic, multimodal, and interactional evidence that support the idea of 2PL referring exclusively to the clients.

In Extract 1, a group of two support workers and ten clients is talking about selecting clients for the Transitional Employment Program, through which the Clubhouse offers supported employment (see Clubhouse International, 2019: Employment programs). One of the support workers (SW1) proposes that the group decides in which of the weekly meetings the selections should be made.

Extract 1

```
01 SW1: me voitas tässä nyt se päättää et kumpiko ryhmä sil
        we could decide it here, which group, it does not

02      ei varmaan oo kauheesti väl[iä et meille käy ainaki
        really matter much, at least we
                         ↑___________________________________
                         ((gazes SW2))

03 SW2:                            [mm.

04 SW1: henkilökunnalle ihan kumpi vaan et
        the staff members are okay with
        __________________________________↑

05      mitä te     ootte  mieltä.
        what you-2PL be-2PL mind-PAR
        what do you think?
             ↑______________↑
             ((gazes O->H->V->S->N->K, see Picture 1 and 2))
```

In Extract 1, SW1 contrasts the expression *meille henkilökunnalle*, "*we, the staff members*" with *te*, "you" making it clear that *you* excludes the staff (*at least we the staff members are okay with either so what do you think*, lines 2 and 4). In the data, there are also cases in which the support workers use an emphasized expression *te **ite***, "you **yourselves**" when referring to the clients, which underlines the demand for their participation in particular (on the functions of 2PL forms, see below).

Referents can also be marked multimodally. Gaze behavior is known to be organized with respect to the sequence organization of courses of action. For example, speakers tend to look at the recipients during question turns in order to solicit a response (Rossano, 2013). Studies have also shown that second-person references in turns that provoke second-pair parts are typically accompanied by gaze (Lerner, 1996; Seppänen, 1998, p. 166). This also applies to our data. In Extract 1, when SW1 is talking about the support workers' opinion, she gazes at SW2, and when she asks for the clients' opinions, she shifts her

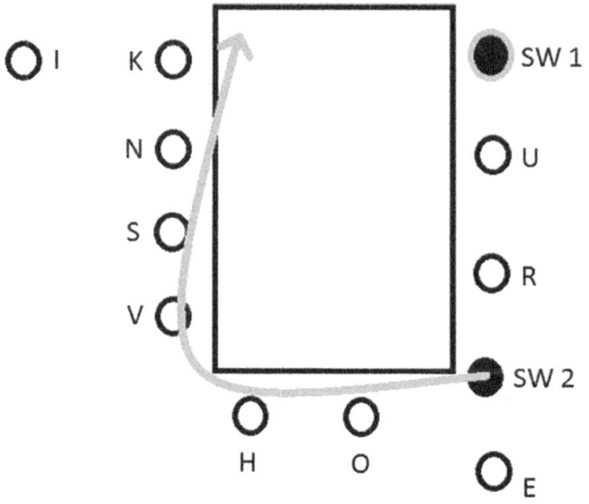

Picture 9.1 Sitting order and SW1's gaze shift (arrow depicts the targets)

gaze from client to client around the table (line 5, see Picture 9.1). Simultaneously, she makes a subtle pointing gesture with her hand up and fingers spread toward the clients (Picture 9.2). In other examples the loosely open hand may also rotate simultaneously with the shifting gaze.

Conclusions about the reference can also be drawn based on turn-taking: who recognize themselves as the referents and reply, and who do not. In our data, it is the clients who reply to the first-pair parts containing 2PL forms—that is, if there is a reply (see Extracts 2–5). Other support workers refrain from producing second-pair parts but may ally with the proposal in other ways. In fact, some of the 2PL references in the proposal sequences are "echoes" of an earlier proposal made by another support worker that has not received uptake from the clients (see below).

To conclude, there is linguistic, embodied, and interactional evidence of the support workers' 2PL references referring to clients and excluding other support workers. Using 2PL as a default reference form for the clients obviously makes the distinction between the support workers and the clients ordinary and unmarked (Enfield, 2007).

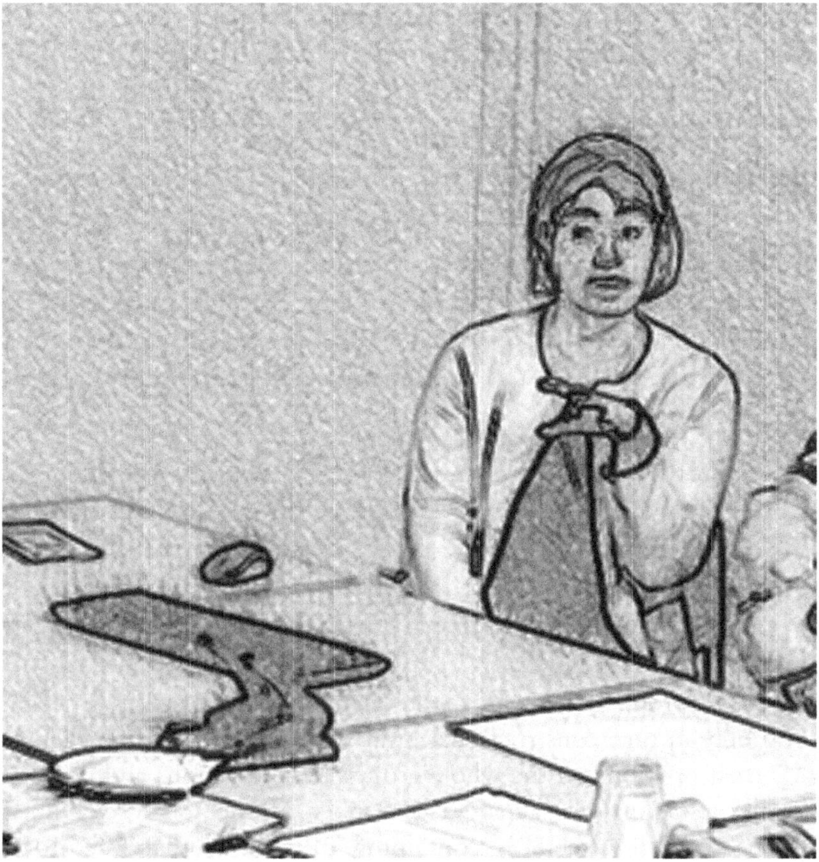

Picture 9.2 Support worker gazing and pointing at clients

Invoking the Distinctiveness of the Client View

Second-person plural forms are often used to ask or tell people to do something, or to evaluate them (Pälli, 2003, pp. 128–130). Our data illustrate the idea of influencing and persuading an outgroup. The support workers' proposals cover a variety of actions, such as organizing meetings, discussing different topics, and filling in forms. However, the verbs the second-person plural forms are used to depict cognitive and emotional actions and speech acts: thinking, desiring, and expressing an opinion (Halliday, 1994).

```
a) mi-tä     te      ajattele-tte  että me
   what-PAR you-2PL think-2PL     CP   we
   what do you think we could
   voitas          ens   kerra-lla tehdä
   can-COND-PASS   next  turn-ADE  do-INF
   do next time.

b) mi-tä     te          toivo-isi-tte käy-
   what-PAR you-2PL (.) wish-COND-2PL (fragment)
   what would you (.) wish
   jatke-taan-ko    tä-stä    keskustelu-a
   continue-PASS-Q this-ELA conversation-PAR
   do we continue discussing
   et mi- mikä tää  siirtymätyö            on,
   CP what     this transition.employment be,
   transitional employment and what it is

c) m-itä     sano-tte.
   what-PAR say-2PL
   what do you say
```

Thus, in proposal sequences, the clients are addressed as a separate group only in turn constructional units explicitly inviting the clients to share their opinions on the whole group's desired actions and decisions. We call these units *view elicitors* (see Reuber, Toerien, Shaw, & Duncan, 2015). Since all utterances containing 2PL forms that refer to the clients are view elicitors in the proposal sequences, referring to the clients as a separate group strongly relates to the effort to enhance client participation in decision-making.

The view elicitors follow established patterns and are used to contextualize or re-contextualize the proposals in a manner that emphasizes the idea of exchanging views rather than seeking for (right) answers. A closer analysis of the sequential context reveals that these view elicitors serve at least two functions: they attract the clients' attention and increase the pressure to contribute to the conversation. In the following, we provide examples of these two functions.

Attracting Attention

Addressing someone in a conversation summons their attention: the addressee is requested to listen to what the speaker has to say (e.g., *Hey, you!*, Lerner, 1996). The 2PL view elicitors in our data are often used as prefaces in proposals. They function as pragmatic markers that highlight thinking and expressing an opinion as the key activities (cf. question frames referring to cognitive actions, Lindström & Lindholm, 2009, pp. 183–193). View elicitors directed to the clients attract their attention and remind them about their chance to influence the decisions. In Extract 2, a support worker (SW2) suggests everybody in the group speak about their former employment.

Extract 2

```
01 SW2: no mitäs ootte sellasesta mieltä et
        well what do you-2PL think about such an idea that
        ↑_______________________________↑↑________________
        ((gazes A))                    ((gazes H and E))

02      jos jokainen haluais esitellä itse
        if everyone would like to present by themselves
        __________↑↑__________________________________
                  ((turns head right and gazes L))

03      oman jonkun työpaikkansa missä on ollu (0.2)
        one of the jobs they have had (0.2)
        ____________________________________________↑

04      kertois siitä vähän laajemmi,
        would tell us about it a bit more broadly.
        ↑___________________________↑↑________↑
        ((turns head left and gazes A))((gazes H))

05      (3.0)

06 Y:   täs ryhmässä.
        in this group.

07 SW2: nii tässä [ryhmässä meille, niinku porukalle
        yes in this group, for us, like for the bunch

08 O:             [hoo hoh hoijaa
                  ((gasp that depicts yawning))

09 Y:   °m mh. m,°
```

In Extract 2, SW2 initiates her turn with a view elicitor (line 1) produced in a colloquial manner. Both the dialog particle *no*, "well," and the tone particle *-s* in ***mitäs*** are typically used in topic-initiating questions, like in our extract. They soften the question and create a friendly "how about" tone (Lindström & Lindholm, 2009, pp. 196–200; Raevaara, 2004). The view elicitor is followed by a proposition, which contains elements that express delicacy (***jos*** *jokainen* ***haluais*** *esitellä*, "**if** everyone **would like** to present"). Talking about a former employment may be challenging for a group of people who have spent some time excluded from the labor market because of mental health difficulties. Thus, complying with the proposition is approached with caution, whereas expressing an opinion about the proposition is treated as effortless.

Indeed, the proposal is received with passive resistance (Stivers, 2007). At first, there is a three-second long silence, followed by client Y's request for clarification (lines 5–6). When SW2 confirms the idea of giving a presentation to the whole group, client O produces a long and articulated gasp depicting the sound of yawning (*hoo hoh hoijaa*, line 8). This client is known for medication-caused fatigue, but this particular gasp can also signal "give me a break" in Finnish. Thus, it is difficult to assess whether O is just expressing the physical experience of being tired or if she finds the proposal tiresome. This is followed by Y producing quiet response particles, signaling understanding of the proposal and perhaps also weak agreement with it (on Finnish response particles, see Sorjonen, 2001).

Our next extract features how SW1 initiates a decision by asking the group if they would like to review the selection criteria for the Transitional Employment program (lines 1–5).

```
Extract 3
01 SW1: mutta mitä ootte nyt mieltä, (0.3) tota (.)
        but now what do you think, (0.3) well (.)

02      halutaanks me nyt niistä enää pikasesti käydä mitään
        do we want to quickly go through any of them

03      läpi (0.3) et mitä ne valinta(0.5)kriteerit tai
        anymore (0.3) what are the selection(0.5)criteria or

04      mi- millä tavalla se siirtymätyöhön lähtijä
        ho- how the person to enter the transitional

05      sitten valitaan siinä yhteisössä?
        employment will be chosen in the community?

06 L:   ni mä ainaki [tykkäisin] (.) että tota
        well at least I would like (.) that erm

07 SW1:              [vai tota ]
                     [or erm   ]

08 L:  [ aih]etta käsiteltäis vähä tota kerrottais
       the subject would be discussed a bit or explained

09 SW1: [ni. ]
        [yes.]

10 SW1: että kun en oo @yht(h)ään@ niinku perehtynyt
        since I have not @at (h)all@ acquainted myself with

11      tähä et, (0.2) enkä oo kertaakaa ollu palaverissa.
        this, (0.2) and have not once attended the meetings.
```

SW1 prefaces her question with a 2PL view elicitor (*mutta mitä **ootte** nyt mieltä*, "but now what do **you** think," but changes the personal reference to 1PL in the question (*halutaanks **me** nyt niistä enää pikasesti käydä mitään läpi*, "do **we** want to quickly go through any of them anymore"). Hence, the clients are asked for their opinion about reviewing the criteria, but they are not expected to do the reviewing by themselves: the clients and support workers will work together as "we" if a review is desired. Thus, the changes in the personal reference mark a shift in perspective.

SW1's question seemingly prefers a negative answer: it contains the negative elements *enää* "anymore" and *mitään* "any, nothing" (line 2), instead of their positive counterparts *vielä* "again, more" and *joitakin* "some." SW1 also appears to attempt to introduce an alternative to reviewing the criteria during client L's turn ("or erm," line 7), but stops and lets L finish her turn. The obvious alternative to reviewing would be proceeding on the agenda. However, as it turns out, this is the first employment coaching meeting for L, and she would therefore like to hear more about the criteria (lines 6, 8, 10–11). Nevertheless, it can be delicate to ask about something that is known to the rest of the group, which is reflected in L's nervous laughter (line 10). In fact, soon after this extract client L herself proposes reading the material later and suggests advancing on the agenda.

In both Extracts 2 and 3, the support workers address the Clubhouse clients using 2PL in the preface of their proposal, attracting their attention. The view elicitor also emphasizes the demand for client participation in terms of interaction: clients are not pressured to consent to what is being proposed but to participate actively in decision-making. This pressuring function seems stronger in cases where the view elicitor is produced later in the proposal sequence. This is demonstrated in the next section.

Pursuing Responses

When someone is addressed in a first-pair part of an adjacency pair, they are also expected to respond by producing the second-pair part (Schegloff & Sacks, 1973). In our data, support workers' 2PL view elicitors are apparently an efficient resource to elicit client participation for exactly this reason. When a view elicitor is produced at an initial or mid-stage of a proposition, it seems to encourage client participation by stressing that the floor is open to hear their opinions, regardless of their thoughts about what is being proposed. However, in cases when the proposition is produced before the clients are addressed, the effect of the view elicitor becomes more imperative.

In Extract 4, the group is creating a poster. SW1 contemplates different poster-making solutions and asks for the group's opinion.

Extract 4

```
01 SW1: millälailla me nyt se askarrellaan sitten että
        how do we now do crafts then like

02      tehääks me tota (0.2) käsin (0.2) pahville
        do we make like (0.2) by hand (0.2) on a cardboard

03      tuol on pahvejaki kyl mitä me voidaan käyttää.
        there is actually some cardboard that we can use.
        ↑________________↑
        ((points and looks to the corner))

04 SW2: m[m.

05 SW1:  [vai onks se sitten et tehdään tietokoneella
         [or is it then that we make it on the computer
                                        ↑_____________↑
                              ((points and looks at screen))

06       ja tulostetaan (0.2) aakolmosta ja,
         and print (0.2) on A3-paper and
                             ↑______________↑
                             ((points and looks at wall))

07      (1.5)

08 SW2: mitä ootte  mieltä
        what be-2PL mind-PAR
        what do you think?
        ↑_________________↑
        ((turns head right and gazes P))

09      (2.0) ((turns head left and gazes E))

10 SW2: miten ois selkeempi.
        how would it be clearer.
        ↑__________↑↑__________↑
 ((gazes E and SW1))((E and SW2 gaze each other))

11 E:   oisko tommoset kartongit kivempiä(h)he(h)
        would those cardboards be nicer (h)he(h)

12 SW2: niin ne on kivempia(h). kyllä.
        yes they are nicer(h). yes.
```

SW1 lists two options: they can either make the poster by hand on colored cardboard or use the printer. Her turn gives the impression of thinking out loud: she gazes around the room, "bites" her index finger, and crinkles her nose ("thinking face," Goodwin & Goodwin, 1986). After a pause and no uptake from the clients, SW2 allies with SW1 and produces a view elicitor that echoes the first-pair part function of SW1's previous turn (*mitä ootte mieltä*, "what do you think," line 8). Her question is followed by silence during which SW2 gazes first at client P, and then at E. In line 10, SW2 reformulates the question (*miten ois selkeempi*, "how would it be clearer"). Client E responds with an evaluation, and SW2 agrees (11–12).

In the next extract, the group is discussing the name of their new weekly meeting. The extract was preceded by several suggestions made by the clients, none of which received notable support. Here, SW3 suggests collecting ideas and then voting.

Extract 5a

```
01 SW3: mitä jos laitetaan sellanen (.) lappu
        what if we would put the kind of (.) note

02      johonki tohon seinälle
        somewhere there on the wall

03      ninku et ehdota nimeä ja äänestetään ja katotaan
        like suggest a name and let's vote and look

04      niistä       [jotenki] sit ens viikolla että mikä
        out of those [somehow] next week like what

05 T:                [↑nii.   ]
                     [↑yeah.  ]

06 SW3: tää on että, (0.2) siihen voi viikon verran kerätä t-
        this is, (0.2) during the week could be collected
```

```
07        keksii ajatuksia tai jotaki sellasta,(1.5)(jotaki)
          come up with ideas or something like that,(1.5)(smth)

08        (.) tai niinku, (.) jos täs on nyt vaikee herätellä
          (.) or like, (.) if it is hard to ponder here and now

09        vai (0.5) vai vai (0.3) mennäänkö valmennusryhmällä?
          or (0.5) or or (0.3) shall we go with coaching group?

10       (3.0)

11 SW3:   se on kyllä kuvaava,
          it is quite fitting,
12 T:     °mm hm°

13        (4.0)

14 SW1:   mitä sanotte.
          what do you say.
          ↑____________↑
          ((looks down on her notepad))

15        (1.0)

16 SW1:   kumpi kampi.
          this or that
          ↑___________↑
          ((starts to write a note))

17 W:     heh

18 T:     no o:nhan se hyvä jos niit on ninku (.)
          well it is certainly good if there are those like (.)

19        seinäl nähtävissä niitä nimiehdotuksia,
          visible on the wall those name suggestions,
```

In Extract 5a, SW3's proposal only evokes a minimal comment from client T (*nii*, "yeah," line 5), so she continues elaborating her idea and suggests another alternative (line 9). In response, the clients remain passive, gazing in an unfocused manner and seemingly avoiding engagement (cf. Goodwin, 1981, p. 98). After a three-second-long silence, SW3 evaluates the suggested name as "fitting," which is weakly agreed to by client T (lines 11–12). Another four seconds pass without any signs of agreement or disagreement. At this moment, SW1 produces the view elicitor *mitä sanotte* "what do you say." By teaming up with SW3, SW1 positions herself as someone who is entitled to pursue answers while withholding her own views—an epitome of an institutional agent.

SW1's contribution is followed by an extended response in which T supports SW3's idea of a vote. However, the other clients remain passive, which appears to jam the conversation. Then, SW3 continues her search for clients' opinions:

Extract 5b

```
22        (4.0)((SW3 turns her head and gazes at clients on
          her right, then looks at T on her left))

23 SW3:   sä       ehdotat   että kysytään
          you-SG2 suggest-2 CP   ask-PASS
          you suggest that we ask

24        (1.0)

25 T:     ↑n::iin on se hy[vä v]armaan nii.
          ↑ye::ah it is go[od I] I guess yea.

26 SW3:                   [nii,]
                          [yea,]

27        (1.5)

28 SW3:   mitä muut sanoo.
          what do the others say.

29        (5.0)((SW3 gazes around))

30 N:     hiljasta on.
          it is silent.

31 SW3:   hiljasta o(h)n. heh näin o,
          silent i(h)t is. heh that's right,
```

Gazing at each client, SW3 reformulates T's previous contribution, and T confirms her understanding (lines 22–25, see Heritage, 1985). After a silence SW3 produces an explicit view elicitor (line 28) referring to the passive participants as *muut*, "the others." This illuminates a common problem of joint decision-making in mental health rehabilitation: a decision cannot be reached jointly unless enough participants express their views, but due to differences in clients' interactional competence and health, the ideal amount of support may be impossible to reach. "The others" may remain passive or choose to withhold their opinion, and in principle, they must be allowed to do so. In Extract 5b, the jammed situation is relieved by humorous comments about the silence (30–31). The sequence ends with the support workers making the decision by themselves (see Extract 4 in Chapter 2), thus compensating for the lack of client participation. Consensus is reached through non-opposition (Urfalino, 2014; see also Chapter 12).

Compared to instances of using a view elicitor during the initial stage of a proposal sequence, a view elicitor that is produced later in the sequence underlines the demand for client participation. However, our data suggest that a pursuit to take a stance during the later stage of the sequence may also be interpreted as a demand to agree (see Extracts 4 and 5a), unlike the view elicitors to attract attention at the beginning of the sequence, in response to which the clients also produce disagreeing turns (Extracts 2 and 3). Prefacing a proposal with a view elicitor evokes the thinking process, while a view elicitor as an independent pursuit for response demands a second-pair part and gives the recipients only little time to cognitive processing (Lindström & Lindholm, 2009).

Discussion: Paradoxes of Inclusion

In this study, we have demonstrated that support workers in mental health rehabilitation address the clients with unmarked second-person plural forms during decision-making sequences. We have shown that the reference to the clients is signaled through verbal and embodied means, and that clients themselves recognize the reference. Furthermore, our analysis indicates that the departures from *us* to *you* are restricted to formulaic view elicitors, whereas the proposed actions are presented from the viewpoint of the whole group. This second-person use highlights the effort to engage clients in interaction and decision-making, which is an important part of the counseling role of the support workers (Trotzer, 1999).

Although addressing the Clubhouse clients as an outgroup can be seen as a practice emphasizing a role division undesired in the Clubhouse model (Chen, 2017), for the same reason it can be an effective means to encourage clients' participation in decision-making. The analysis revealed that direct invitations to share a view in combination with embodied inclusion evoke client participation, as these practices attract attention and make participation both relevant and anticipated. Paradoxically, inclusion is achieved by using a practice that entails an apparent element of exclusion. By addressing clients as a separate group, support workers refrain from speaking on everyone's behalf, and thus decrease their own power of decision to some extent. Using 2PL view-elicitors is a way to construct a shared understanding at the meetings.

Our further analysis demonstrates that the form of participation may be affected by the sequential placement of the 2PL view elicitor. Using a view elicitor as a part of a multi-unit turn (as a preface or a final turn-constructional unit) seems to encourage clients to share their thoughts, while an independent view elicitor produced after a pause may be treated as a demand to agree. From this viewpoint, the lack of client response may not only be a sign of indifference or disengagement but a form of rebellion against the expectation to accept the support workers' initiatives. Thus, the act of not participating explicitly in a decision-making sequence could be regarded as a statement or an effort to hinder the modus operandi used in the meetings. These actions of avoidance are comparable to leaving an empty vote or not voting in an election. These choices both disturb making a democratic decision and express sovereignty and bring forward the threat that is the tyranny of the majority (see Saunders, 2008). However, as our data reveal, the absence of explicit agreements and disagreements slows down the decision-making process but does not halt it; the support workers may harness their institutional power and decide by themselves in order to proceed the meeting (see also Karlsson, 2005; Valkeapää et al., 2018).

All in all, the planning of future Clubhouse activities is obviously controlled by the support workers, and the clients who participate in interaction actively are likely to succumb to what is recommended by the staff. However, the idea of the more competent and active participants compensating for the less competent or disengaged ones is not necessarily in contradiction with the Clubhouse's recovery approach and its emphasis on individual progress (Anthony, 2007). In addition to individual abilities, there are individual limitations, and they both need to be met with respect. Nevertheless, the communal ideology of the Clubhouse emerges in the support workers' efforts to provide the clients with recognizable opportunities for contribution. This conduct recognizes the clients as valuable resources who are not there only to be helped but also to help each other and the whole group (Trotzer, 1999).

Based on our findings we believe that training support workers to be more aware of the inevitable role division between the staff and the clients would be beneficial for joint decision-making. Raising the awareness of interactional power relations could help them use their institutional stance in a way that promotes inclusion but does not burden the clients to excess. For example, support workers could be encouraged to address the clients explicitly when making decisions about activities that concern them. Embedding an open call for the clients' views, such as *What do you think?* in a proposal turn highlights the opportunity to contribute if and when ready.

References

Anthony, W. A. (2007). *Toward a vision of recovery: For mental health and psychiatric rehabilitation services*. Boston: Boston University Press.

Chen, F. (2017). Building a working community: Staff practices in a Clubhouse for people with severe mental illness. *Administration and Policy in Mental Health, 44*(5), 651–663.

Clubhouse International. (2019). http://clubhouse-intl.org.

Drew, P., & Heritage, J. (Eds.). (1992). *Talk at work: Interaction in institutional settings*. Cambridge: Cambridge University Press.

Enfield, N. J. (2007). Meanings of the unmarked: How "default" person reference does more than just refer. In T. Stivers & N. J. Enfield (Eds.), *Person reference in interaction: Linguistic, cultural and social perspectives* (pp. 97–120). New York: Cambridge University Press.

Goffman, E. (1981). *Forms of talk*. Pennsylvania: University of Pennsylvania Press.

Goodwin, C. (1981). *Conversational organization: Interaction between speakers and hearers*. New York: Academic Press.

Goodwin, M., & Goodwin, C. (1986). Gesture and coparticipation in the activity of searching for a word. *Semiotica, 62*(1–2), 51–76.

Halliday, M. A. K. (1994). *An introduction to functional grammar*. London: Edward Arnold.

Hänninen, E. (2012). *Choices for recovery: Community-based rehabilitation and the Clubhouse model as means to mental health reforms*. Helsinki: Finnish Institute for Health and Welfare.

Helasvuo, M.-L., & Laitinen, L. (2006). Person in Finnish: Paradigmatic and syntagmatic relations in interaction. In M.-L. Helasvuo & L. Campbell (Eds.), *Grammar from the human perspective: Case, space and person in Finnish* (pp. 173–207). Amsterdam: Benjamins.

Heritage, J. (1985). Analyzing news interviews: Aspects of the production of talk for an "overhearing" audience. In T. Van Dijk (Ed.), *Handbook of discourse analysis* (pp. 95–119). London: Academic Press.

Hickey, G., & Kipping, C. (1998). Exploring the concept of user involvement in mental health through a participation continuum. *Journal of Clinical Nursing, 7*(1), 83–88.

Karlsson, M. (2005). Fountain house. In T. Borkman, M. Karlsson, C. Munn-Giddings, & L. Smith (Eds.), *Self-help and mental health: Case studies of mental health self-help organizations in US, England and Sweden* (pp. 95–106). Stockholm: Sköndalsinstitutets Research Department.

Lerner, G. (1993). Collectivities in action: Establishing the relevance of conjoined participation in conversation. *Interdisciplinary Journal for the Study of Discourse, 13*(2), 213–246.

Lerner, G. (1996). On the place of linguistic resources in the organization of talk-in-interaction: 'Second person' reference in multi-party conversation. *Pragmatics, 6,* 281–294.

Lindström, J., & Lindholm, C. (2009). "May I ask!": Question frames in institutional interaction. In M. Haakana, M. Laakso, & J. Lindström (Eds.), *Talk in interaction: Comparative dimensions* (pp. 180–205). Helsinki: Finnish Literature Society.

Pälli, P. (2003). *Ihmisryhmä diskurssissa ja diskurssina* [Human group in discourse and as discourse, English abstract]. Tampere: University of Tampere.

Raevaara, L. (2004). Mitäs me sovittais? *s*-partikkelin sisältävien hakukysymysten tehtävistä. *Virittäjä, 108,* 531–558.

Reuber, M., Toerien, M., Shaw, R., & Duncan, R. (2015). *Delivering patient choice in clinical practice: A conversation analytic study of communication practices used in neurology clinics to involve patients in decision-making.* Southampton, UK: NIHR Journals Library. https://www.ncbi.nlm.nih.gov/books/NBK279940/.

Rossano, F. (2013). Gaze in conversation. In J. Sidnell & T. Stivers (Eds.), *Handbook of conversation analysis* (pp. 308–329). Chichester: Wiley-Blackwell.

Royal College of Psychiatrists Social Inclusion Scoping Group. (2009). *Mental health and social inclusion: Making psychiatry and mental health services fit for the 21st century.* Position Statement PS01/2009. https://www.rcpsych.ac.uk/docs/default-source/mental-health/work-and-mental-health-library/position-statement-2009.pdf?sfvrsn=97bca29e_2.

Sacks, H., & Schegloff, E. A. (1979). Two preferences in the organization of reference to persons in conversation and their interaction. Re-print in T. Stivers & N. J. Enfield (Eds.). (2007). *Person reference in interaction: Linguistic, cultural and social perspectives* (pp. 23–28). New York: Cambridge University Press.

Sacks, H., Schegloff, E. A., & Jefferson, G. (1974). A simplest systematics for the organization of turn-taking for conversation. *Language, 50*(4), 696–735.

Saunders, B. (2008). *Democracy-as-fairness: Justice, equal chances, and lotteries.* PhD thesis. Department of Politics and International Relations, University of Oxford. https://web.archive.org/web/20080910032028/http://oxford.academia.edu/documents/BenSaunders_SubmittedThesis.pdf.

Schegloff, E. A. (1996). Some practices of referring to persons in talk-in-interaction: A partial sketch of a systematics. In B. Fox (Ed.), *Studies in anaphora* (pp. 437–485). Amsterdam: Benjamins.

Schegloff, E. A., & Sacks, H. (1973). Opening up closings. *Semiotica, 8*(4), 69–99.

Seppänen, E.-L. (1998). *Läsnäolon pronominit: Tämä, tuo, se ja hän viittaamassa keskustelun osallistujaan* [Pronouns of participation: The Finnish pronouns tämä, tuo, se and hän as devices for referring to co-participants in conversation, English abstract]. Helsinki: Finnish Literature Society.

Sidnell, J., & Stivers, T. (Eds.). (2013). *Handbook of conversation analysis.* Chichester: Wiley-Blackwell.

Sorjonen, M.-L. (2001). *Responding in conversation: A study of response particles in Finnish*. Amsterdam: Benjamins.
Stivers, T. (2007). *Prescribing under pressure: Parent-physician conversations and antibiotics*. Oxford: Oxford University Press.
Suomalainen, K. (2018). *Sinä*, konteksti ja monitulkintaisuus: Yksikön 2. persoonan viittaukset arkikeskustelussa [*Sinä* 'you', context, and ambiguity: Second-person singular reference in everyday Finnish conversation, English abstract]. *Virittäjä, 122*(3), 320–355.
Tajfel, H. (1981). *Human groups and social categories: Studies in social psychology*. Cambridge: Cambridge University Press.
Trotzer, J. (1999). *The counselor and the group: Integrating theory, training, and practice*. New York: Taylor & Francis.
Urfalino, P. (2014). The rule of non-opposition: Opening up decision-making by consensus. *Journal of Political Philosophy, 22*(3), 320–341.
Valkeapää, T., Tanaka, K., Lindholm, C., Weiste, E., & Stevanovic, M. (2018). Interaction, ideology, and practice in mental health rehabilitation. *Journal of Psychosocial Rehabilitation and Mental Health, 6*(1), 9–23.

10

Co-constructing Desired Activities: Small-Scale Activity Decisions in Occupational Therapy

Elina Weiste

Enabling Client Participation Through Therapeutic Collaboration

Current international mental health policy recommendations emphasize the importance of client participation (WHO, 2010). Research has shown that clients' active participation can be increased by a client-centered service model that tailors support to clients' individual needs and promotes their skills and confidence (e.g., Hibbard & Greene, 2013). The core idea of this model is to elicit and understand clients' perspectives, expectations, and needs in order to reach a shared understanding of the problem and its treatment, as well as to help clients share power and responsibility by involving them in decision-making (Epstein et al., 2005, p. 1517). In shared decision-making, both parties share information and take steps to construct a joint view on the preferred treatment (Charles, Gafnv, & Whelan, 1997).

E. Weiste (✉)
Finnish Institute of Occupational Health, Helsinki, Finland
e-mail: elina.weiste@ttl.fi

C. Lindholm et al. (eds.), *Joint Decision Making in Mental Health*,
The Language of Mental Health, https://doi.org/10.1007/978-3-030-43531-8_10

The shared decision-making paradigm largely focuses on describing high-stakes decision-making: situations concerning treatment decisions that have a significant impact on the client's life (see Chapters 3, 5, and 7 in this volume). However, operating within a client-centered framework also necessitates considering decision-making opportunities in "smaller," more everyday areas of life (see also Chapters 2, 6, 8, 10, and 12). Even though these small-scale decisions might lack the kind of consequentiality that characterizes treatment decisions, they are nevertheless considered important for taking the client's perspective into account and supporting the client's progress (e.g., Sumsion, 2006). This is especially the case with clients with severe mental illnesses, such as schizophrenia, which are known to impair clients' decision-making capacity (e.g., Beitinger, Kissling, & Hamann, 2014).

However, previous research has not investigated how this small-scale decision-making is realized in interaction. This chapter complements previous research on shared decision-making by exploring the way the therapist and client make small-scale decisions during occupational therapy sessions. It focuses on proposals made by the occupational therapists and clients while engaged in shared activities that are meaningful to the client.

Meaningful Activities as Therapeutic Interventions

Participating in different forms of activities is fundamental to human health and well-being. Such activities provide meaning and structure to people's lives, are important in the development of identity, and reflect society's values and culture (Creek, 2014; WFOT, 2012). The aim of occupational therapy is to promote, maintain, or restore clients' well-being and functional independence through meaningful activities (*occupations*) that the clients wish to perform (WFOT, 2012). The primary goal is to enable clients to participate in the activities of everyday life: taking care of themselves, managing domestic life, coping at school and work, resting, spending leisure time, and participating in society. The therapeutic process is set to foster the client's sense of belonging and connecting to others through participation in activities that are valued in the client's social context and have potential to strengthen his or her social roles (Hammell, 2014). This therapeutic goal is achieved by working with clients to enhance their ability to engage in the activities that they wish, need, or are expected to perform or by modifying those activities or the environment to better support their engagement (WFOT, 2012).

Occupational therapists often use different types of activities meaningful to the client as therapeutic tools for precipitating changes in the client's function and performance (Creek, 2014). The *desired activity* is the task or occupation that the therapist and client have selected for therapy (Taylor, 2008, p. 53). Clients are actively involved in the therapeutic process, and the general goal of the interventions is to increase the client's occupational performance and develop skills to support health, well-being, and life satisfaction (WFOT, 2012).

In an occupational therapy process, a therapist and client engage in activities that they perform collaboratively during the therapeutic sessions. An important part of this joint performance involves providing clients with the opportunity to make small-scale decisions on the activities they wish to perform (e.g., Creek, 2014; Taylor, 2008). These *activity decisions* are deliberate decisions that concern what the therapist and client will do together during their joint session, usually in the following minutes (Kielhofner, 2002).

This chapter investigates how small-scale activity decisions are jointly constructed by occupational therapists and clients. The analysis focuses on the proposals that participants make while performing an activity selected by the client, such as cooking or artwork, during the therapy session. Proposals are acts of speech in which one of the participant's names a forward-looking act and suggests its implementation—proposing it to others for confirmation or rejection (Stevanovic, 2012). Proposals are of interest from the perspective of therapeutic collaboration, as participants assign their partner-in-interaction equal status to decide on future activities (Stevanovic, 2012).

Research Questions

The aim in this chapter is to complement previous work on shared decision-making by exploring the proposals therapists and clients make while engaged in a joint activity. The analysis is guided by the following research questions:

1. What proposals do occupational therapists and clients make when engaged in a joint activity?
2. What verbal and material resources do therapists and clients use in their proposals?
3. How are these proposals sequentially located as part of the activity performance?

Data and Method

The data consist of 15 video-recordings of occupational therapy encounters in Finland, collected from two different psychiatric outpatient clinics. In Finland, psychiatric outpatient clinics provide psychiatric consultation, treatment, and rehabilitation for the adult population of the local community. A referral from a primary care doctor is needed. A broad range of acute and chronic mental disorders is treated, and the services provided to the client free of charge.

The length of the therapy sessions varies from 45 minutes to two hours and comprises 16 hours of interaction. The data come from three therapists with three different clients. The therapists are all qualified occupational therapists and the clients all suffer from severe mental illnesses, such as schizophrenia, schizoaffective disorder, and major depression. At the time of the data collection, they were engaged in ongoing therapeutic relationships that had lasted from six months to two years. Their regular meetings were held at approximately two-week intervals. Permission to collect the data was obtained from the municipal health authority and the ethical board of the University

Central Hospital. All names and other details which could enable identification of the participants have been altered in the data extracts.

From the dataset, the sessions selected were those in which the participants engaged in joint activities. From the entire set of 16 sessions, four contained such activity-oriented sessions, during which the clients cooked and practiced several types of art. The data were analyzed by means of conversation analysis (e.g., Sidnell & Stivers, 2013). In the analytic procedure (see e.g., Heritage, 2011), the recordings were first listened to several times, and then all the instances in which the therapist or the client made a proposal while engaged in a joint activity were selected. Other proposals outside the immediate activity context, such as decisions on what activities to perform during the sessions, were excluded from this analysis. The dataset contained 31 such small-scale decision-making sequences. In what follows, the therapeutic functions of these decision-making sequences are investigated in detail, focusing on their consequences for the subsequent interaction.

Constructing a Shared Activity Through Small-Scale Decisions

The analysis reveals that the occupational therapists performed two types of interactional work. First, they made room for the clients' proposals by shaping the activity context. They invited clients' proposals by noticing resources or materials and making them publicly visible. They also described their own actions and possible problems relating to the objects, making it relevant for the client to propose solutions or subsequent activity steps. Second, the occupational therapists made proposals themselves. They were used to suggest the order of activity steps or the ways the performance should be achieved. Thus, these proposals worked primarily as an aid or support for the client's occupational performance. In the following, each of these two types of proposals is illustrated through data examples.

Enabling Client Proposals by Shaping the Activity Context

In the present data, the therapists implicitly invited the clients to make proposals by shaping the activity context. The first practice that the therapists used to invite client's proposals was to notice materials in the therapy room. By making physical objects publicly visible, the therapist invited the client to propose how to use them in order to proceed with the activity at hand. Extract 1 provides a case in point.

In Extract 1, the client (C) and therapist (T) have been discussing the client's anxiety attacks, and they have sought ways to manage them. They have agreed to make a note card that the client can use when feeling distressed in public spaces. Just before the extract occurs, they have written the text that will be on the card, and the therapist, who is using a computer, begins to modify the size of the text.

Extract 1

01 T: minkä kokosen sinä tästä halusit (.) oliko tää
what size did you want this to be (.) was it

02 lom [pakkoon
for [your wallet ((T gazes computer))

03 C: [joo lompakkokoko eli tota (0.5) ehkä niinku
[yes wallet size so erm (0.5) maybe erm

04 valkoselle pohjalle tai (0.2) tota,
the background or (0.2) erm,

05 T: hei mulla on tuossa sitten tuo ↑printteri,
hey then I have that ↑printer over there,
↑________________↑ ↑__________________↑
((T gazes C)) ((T points at the printer))

06 C: **↑joo (.) joo pitäskö se eka niinku tulostaa ja kattoo**
↑yes (.) yes should we first print it out and see

07 **että [mahtuuko se sitte.**
if it[fits then.

08 T: [joo tuloste[taa::npas.
[yes let's print it ou::t ((turns towards the computer))

The therapist asks for the client's preferences over the size of the text to be printed on the card (line 1). The therapist also checks if the client's plan was to put the note card in her wallet. The client agrees and confirms that the card should be "wallet size" (line 3), but she has difficulty identifying the size of the text. The client hesitates, pauses her speech, and tells the therapist to use "a white background" (line 4), thereby failing to respond to the therapist's initial question about the size of the text. In line 5, the therapist makes a notable departure from the previous turns of talk: the turn is initiated with the interjection *hei* ("hey"), which seeks to focus the client's attention (Hakulinen et al., 2004, § 858). It is followed by a statement in which the therapist notes that she has a printer on her side-desk. She also turns her gaze from the computer toward the client and points at the printer with her index finger. The printer has been there all the time, but at this point, when the object becomes interactionally relevant, she foregrounds it and makes it publicly visible (see Bergmann, 1990). In this way, the therapist provides an implicit hint to the client about how she could solve the problem of text size. In lines 6–7, the client exploits the therapist's hint and proposes that they print the text to see if the size is right. Still overlapping with the client's talk, the therapist agrees, turns toward the computer and starts to print the document (line 8).

In summary, the therapist closely monitors the client's actions, notices a physical object and makes it publicly visible, directing the client's perception toward the object. This provides the client with an implicit hint on how to proceed with the activity at hand. Rather than proposing a solution herself, the therapist gives the client an opportunity to solve the problem and decide how to continue with the activity.

The therapists also shape the preconditions for clients making proposals by describing their own actions related to physical objects and the possible problems therein. In this way, they make it relevant for the client to propose solutions and the next activity steps. Extract 2 provides one such example.

Prior to the extract, the therapist and client have been making refrigerator magnets with supportive messages. At the beginning of the extract, they are starting to glue the text tags into the magnets.

Extract 2

```
01 T: se oli se missä on se piste niin se on se mihin
      it was that dot that is the place you

02    laitetaan liima.
      put the glue.

03 C: joo.
      yes. ((T grasps the bottle of glue))

04 T: mä testaan toimiiko tää liima (1.5) täällä on liimaa
      I'll see if this glue works (1.5) there is some glue
      ↑__________________________________________________↑
      ((T squeezes the glue))

05    mutta tää on ihan tukossa,
      but it is completely clogged up,

06    (2.5) ((T gazes C))

07 T: mä laitan ton (1.7) mä vähän testaan jos tota,
      I'll put that (1.7) I test a bit if erm,
      ↑__________________________________________________↑
      ((T takes a stick and pushes it into the flask))

08 C: mhhh::

09 T: joo mä laitan ton (0.2) mut ei tää näytä auttavan,
      yeah I'll put that (0.2) this doesn't seem to help,
                                  ↑____________________↑
                                  ((T gazes C))

10 C: niin nyt pitäskö ottaa käyttöön toi uudempi keltanen,
      so should we now use that newer yellow one,
                        ↑_______↑
                        ((C points at another bottle of glue))

11 T: no joo ei kai tää (0.2) joo,
      well yeah this isn't (0.2) sure,
```

In lines 1–2, the therapist instructs the client on how to glue the magnets, but when she grasps the bottle of glue, she notices that there is a problem: the glue seems to have dried up. The therapist tries to solve the problem by squeezing the bottle (line 4) and opening it with a stick (line 7). The therapist also uses meta-talk to describe what she is doing (lines 4–5, 7, and 9), although her actions are clearly visible to the client, who is sitting facing the therapist. Moreover, in line 9, the therapist states that her actions seem to have been unsuccessful. She also gazes at the client, offering her a slot to interfere and propose a more successful solution that would enable the progress of the activity. In line 10, the client makes such an inference and proposes that they use the other bottle of glue on the table.

Thus, while the therapist manipulates the object that can be used to solve the problem, she does not perform the whole action and overcome the problem herself. Rather, she describes her own activity steps and unsuccessful attempts and gazes at the client to invite her to participate.

In summary, therapists make room for the client's proposals by shaping the activity context. This is achieved by (1) making physical objects or materials publicly visible and/or (2) describing their own actions relating to problems with the physical objects. In both cases, in our data, the therapist does not bring the desired activity to closure by herself; rather, she provides the client with hints on how to solve the problem and opportunities to decide how to continue.

Therapists' Proposals Supporting the Client's Performance

In addition to inviting clients' proposals, occupational therapists also make proposals themselves during small-scale activity decisions. These proposals suggest the order of the activity steps or the ways the performance should be achieved. Thus, these proposals work primarily as an aid or support for the client's performance. Extract 3 provides an example of a case in which the client is highly agitated, and the therapist's proposals guide her to focus on the activity at hand.

In Extract 3, the therapist and client are cooking. Before the extract occurs, they have agreed to make vegetable soup and read through the recipe. At the beginning of the extract, as they are taking out the ingredients, the client suddenly begins to talk about and show the items that she has bought from the grocery store. The client talks very fast, using unclear references, and it is difficult to follow the relationship between the things she is discussing.

Extract 3

```
01 C: >sitten mä ostin tota mä ostin uuden tämmösen kun se<
      >then I bought erm I bought this new thing when it<

02    oli euro viiskymment niin >mä otin sitte et aattelin et
      was one euro fifty >I took it then then I thought that

03    vähän jos laittas< (.) mä meen nyt kaupan kautta ni
      what if I put some< (.) I'll go to the store then

04    sitten kotiin mutta mul on täällä nyt sitten on näitä,
      before I go home but but now I got these here,

05 T: su[l on,
      you[ have,

06 C:   [näit juttuja et oon miettiny niitä aisteja ja
        [these things so I've thought about those senses and

07    nyt mä en tiiä oikein et miten jaksan mutta,
      now I don't really know that how I'll handle that but,

08 T: no hei   tehdään[kö tuota eka,
      well hey should [we do that first,
                         ↑_______↑
                         ((points at the soup ingredients))

09 C:                  [ja sitte oon suunnitellu vähä tos mä
                       [and then I've planned a bit I

10    en tiedä että,
      don't know that,

11 T: joo-o ni tehdäänkö toi nyt ensiksi.
      yes so should we do that now first.
         ↑______________________↑
         ((smiles and nods towards the soup ingredients))
```

12 C: joo (.) joo ja tota (2.0) ja (0.2) ja .hhhhh
yes (.) yes and erm (2.0) and (0.2) and .hhhhh

13 T: mm niin.

14 C: jos vaikka nyt ih- anteeks kun mä oon näin
if erm ih- I'm so sorry that I'm so

15 hirveen hermostunu.
awfully nervous.

16 T: ei se haittaa °ihan rauhassa°.
it doesn't matter °take it easy°.

17 C: **oliks tää siis ekana,**
was this the first thing,
↑___________↑
((picks up a food item))

In line 1, the client, who has taken the soup ingredients from the closet, turns toward her own bag, takes out a small package of spices, and announces that she bought it because it cost only €1.50. However, it is unclear if the client is proposing that the spice be added to the soup when she asks, "what if I put some?" (line 3). It is also unclear how going to the store after the therapy meeting (lines 3–4) is related to the story or the activity at hand. The client also uses an unclear reference when talking about "these things" (lines 4 and 6) without explaining what they are. In line 5, the therapist initiates a clarifying turn ("you have"), but the client continues her account, overlapping with the therapist's talk. The client now begins to talk about "senses" (line 6), which are seemingly unrelated to anything that has been discussed during the session. She refers to these senses as something she is unable to handle (line 7).

At this point, the therapist takes a turn and makes a proposal. She points at the soup ingredients and suggests the activity order—what they could do "first" (line 8). The client, however, continues once more with her account, again overlapping with the therapist's talk (lines 9–10). In line 11, the therapist proposes for a second time that they first make the soup. She smiles and nods toward the soup ingredients, giving the impression that she is gently guiding the client toward the activity at hand. The client hesitates, inhales deeply (line 12), and apologizes for being in such a nervous state (lines 14–15). After that, the client refocuses on the food items on the table and continues the activity. In line 17, the client presents herself as an active agent who understands the therapist's proposal and accepts it.

Thus, in cases in which the client is agitated or faces other challenges in focusing on the activity at hand, therapist proposals that suggest the order of the activity steps can assist the client's performance. These proposals seem to invite clients' participation and provide them with an opportunity to be active agents who are in control of their own activity performance. These proposals also created an interactional environment in which topics other than issues relating to the activity performance could be raised and discussed. This is demonstrated in Extract 4.

Extract 4 is from a later part of the same session from which Extract 1 was drawn. Here, the therapist has printed the text they are planning to place on the card, which they have slightly modified (see Chapter 8 in this volume on writing in decision-making). In line 1, the therapist and client are looking at the printed text, and the therapist asks if the client is satisfied with it.

Extract 4

```
01 T: ootko sä tyytyväinen tähän fonttiin ja kokoon?
      are you happy with this font and size?

02 C: joo olen olen.
      yes I am I am. ((T turns towards the computer))

03 T: eli nyt tää on korjattu ja sit mä tulostan sulle uuden.
      so now this is fixed and I'll print you a new one.

04 C: juu se on ihan bra,
      yes that is fine,

05 T: joo (0.5) katotaas
      yes (0.5) let's see ((T prints the piece of paper))

06    (3.5) ((T gives the paper to C; C reads it))

07 C: siinä loppupääs (.) ei ei voimiaan säästä varmaan
      at the end (.) it probably doesn't save your strength
      ↑_______________________________________________↑
      ((C gazes the paper))

08    tää et kiskaisee niin ku eteenpäin.
      that you like yank forward
                        ↑_____________↑
                        ((C gazes T))
```

09 T: joo mitä sä haluat siihen laittaa,
yes so what would you like have in there,

10 C: joo ei mitään (.) ei mitään.
yes nothing (.) nothing.

11 (1.5)

12 C: mä just niin ku sillon (.) nyt (0.2) nyt mul on ollu
I just back then (.) now (0.2) now I have been

13 vähän niin kun stressi ja vähä huonompi olo mutta (0.2)
stressed and felt a bit bad but (0.2)

14 tai aika huono (.) siis tosi huono olo.
or pretty bad (.) I mean very bad.

15 (2.0)

16 T: **okei tehäänkö niin et mä oon ny- (0.2) katotaanko tätä**
okay so should we do so that I'm ny-(0.2) should we

17 **vielä ihan ajan kanssa,**
still look at this over time,

18 C: juu juu,
yeah,

19 T: °mmm° mistä sä luulet että se huono olo on johtunut.
°mmm° what do you think causes the bad feeling.

In line 1, the therapist asks if the client is happy with the text, and she also announces that the text has been corrected according to the client's wishes, thereby seemingly treating the text as ready. First in line 2 and then in line 4, the client confirms that she is happy with the text. In line 5, the therapist prints out the piece of paper and gives it to the client. When reading it, the client highlights some parts of the text ("doesn't save your strength," line 7 and "yank forward," line 8) without explaining if or how she wants to correct them. At the end of line 8, the client also turns her gaze from the piece of paper to the therapist, seemingly waiting for her to respond. The therapist orients to the client's turns as a request to change the text and asks how the client would like to modify it (line 9). In line 10, the client nonetheless withdraws, saying that she wants "nothing." After a silence in line 11, the client continues by starting to describe how she has felt stressed and bad. She also upgrades her description from feeling "a bit bad" (line 13) to "pretty bad" and eventually to "very bad" (line 14). At this point, the therapist proposes that they look at the text "over time" (lines 16–17), thus reducing the pace of the activity performance. The client agrees (line 18), and the therapist then asks more about the reasons for the client's feelings of distress. Thus, while still performing the activity at hand, the therapist focuses the talk on the client's feelings.

In addition to helping the client focus on the activity at hand (Extract 3), the therapist can also use proposals to create an interactional environment in which other topics, such as the client's difficult emotional experiences, can be discussed (Extract 4). Thus, therapists' proposals seem to work as an aid for supporting the client's performance and management of the activity at hand.

Discussion

The analysis revealed that occupational therapists perform two types of interactional work when inviting the client's participation in small-scale activity decisions. First, they make room for the client's proposals by shaping the activity context. In my data, they invited the client's proposals by noticing materials and making them publicly visible (Extract 1) and by describing their own actions related to problems with the physical objects (Extract 2). Therefore, the therapists exploited physical, mutable objects as a part of the decision-making sequence (see Fasulo & Monzoni, 2009). Here, the therapists did not complete the activity themselves; rather, they used objects to hint at how to solve the problem and decide how to continue. In this way, they were able to enhance client participation *and* the progression of the activity at hand.

Second, in addition to inviting the client's proposals, the therapists also made proposals themselves. The proposals were used to suggest the order of activity steps or the ways the performance should be achieved (Extract 3). By closely monitoring the client's occupational performance and proposing the order of activity steps, the therapist could facilitate the client's engagement in the activity and help her focus on the activity at hand (see Taylor, 2008). In sum, the analysis demonstrated that clients were provided decision-making power over the substantial matters of the activity, whereas therapists used decision-making power to assist the client's occupational performance and manage the progression of the activity at hand.

The therapists also used proposals to create an interaction environment in which talks could be centered on the client's current feelings (Extract 4). In such cases, the proposals subtly guided the focus of the talk away from the activity. Thus, although they continued to perform the activity, the proposal reduced the pace of the performance, thereby providing the therapist with an opportunity to concentrate on the client's current emotional experience.

Thus, it seems that even though the therapist invited the client to make activity decisions, the goal was not an end-product and a change in the environment caused by the action (Parsons, 1937); rather, the action was seen as a goal in itself (e.g., Arendt, 1958). Extracts 3 and 4 also shows how the therapist's proposals can serve as an arena in which the emotional reactions that stem from and influence the client's occupational engagement can be managed. The therapists' proposals are a momentary locus of interaction where the client's emotions and its implications for occupational participation can be addressed (see Taylor, 2008).

In the present dataset, imperfections and problems during the activities provided possible decision-making moments, with a slowing of the pace of the activity creating the opportunity to decide how to proceed. In Extract 1, the client had difficulty solving a problem related to the size of the piece of paper. The therapist did not rush to solve the problem but offered the client a clue that enabled the client to suggest a way forward. In Extract 2, the therapist made her own difficulty visible and thus offered the client an opportunity to propose a solution. The therapist positioned herself as unknowledgeable, thereby allowing the client to share responsibility and increasing the client's power to decide how to proceed (see Epstein et al., 2005; Weiste, Voutilainen, & Peräkylä, 2016). In this way, clients' active involvement in the therapeutic processes is supported, and they are encouraged to adopt the role of experts in the activity they are performing (Sumsion, 2006; Weiste, 2018). The therapists' practices also revealed a rehabilitative approach, whereby the therapists avoided completing activities in which difficulties were encountered and instead helped clients to find a way to act and resolve the situation themselves (see WFOT, 2012).

The findings highlight the ideal of a reciprocal relationship between the therapist and client (see Harra, 2014). Shared activity allows both parties to adopt the role of equal actors in addition to those of a client and a professional (Harra, 2014). Equality can also be constructed through interaction, by explicitly expressing views about future activities as proposals. A proposal compared to a request or announcement situates both parties in the interaction as equal to decide on future action (Stevanovic, 2012).

But then again, therapists explicitly compensate for their clients' inabilities by supporting client participation and creating decision-making opportunities. The decisions are small enough to be considered the "small agency" described by Honkasalo (2013), where the agency is constructed as a starting point for clients to become still and even tolerate their present situation. When a client is too ill or disabled to participate fully in the therapeutic process, the therapist may have to take responsibility for decision-making, remaining aware of the risk of imposing their own goals and values (Creek, 2014, p. 33). One of the goals of occupational therapy will then be to work toward increasing client understanding, autonomy and choice (Creek, 2014). Thus, for clients with severe and chronic mental health problems, even such small-scale decisions can be important from the perspective of respecting their self-determination and allowing them to express their own will (e.g., Sumsion, 2006). This is also thought to teach clients the skills needed to make decisions that are considerably more significant, such as treatment decisions, which are related to the clients' own care (e.g., Taylor, 2008; see also Chapter 2 in this volume).

As my data demonstrated, joint desired action and therapists' proposals in particular are also used to achieve therapeutic goals, such as structuring the client's occupational performance. Here, therapists use their decision-making power to assist the client's performance but provide the client with opportunities to make the decision concerning the content of the activity. Thus, although the therapeutic relationship can never be completely equal, these practices enable the client to be considered an active subject rather than the object of the professional's performance.

References

Arendt, H. (1958). *The human condition*. Chicago: University of Chicago Press.

Beitinger, R., Kissling, W., & Hamann, J. (2014). Trends and perspectives of shared decision-making in schizophrenia and related disorders. *Current Opinion in Psychiatry, 27*(3), 222–229.

Bergmann, J. (1990). On the local sensitivity of conversation. In I. Markovà & K. Foppa (Eds.), *The dynamics of dialogue* (pp. 201–226). Hemel Hempstead: Harvester.

Charles, C., Gafnv, A., & Whelan, T. (1997). Shared decision-making in the medical encounter: What does it mean? (or it takes at least two to tango). *Social Science and Medicine, 44*(5), 681–692.

Creek, J. (2014). The knowledge base of occupational therapy. In W. Bryant, J. Fieldhouse, & K. Bannigan (Eds.), *Creek's occupational therapy and mental health* (pp. 27–47). Edinburgh: Elsevier.

Epstein, R. M., Franks, P., Fiscella, K., Cleveland, G. S., Meldrum, S. C., Kravitz, R.L., & Duberstein, P. R. (2005). Measuring patient-centred communication in patient-physician consultations: Theoretical and practical issues. *Social Science and Medicine, 61*(7), 1516–1528.

Fasulo, A., & Monzoni, C. (2009). Assessing mutable objects: A multimodal analysis. *Research on Language and Social Interaction, 42*(4), 362–376.

Hakulinen, A., Vilkuna, M., Korhonen, R., Koivisto, V., Heinonen, T. R., & Alho, I. (2004). Iso suomen kielioppi. [Extensive Finnish grammar] Helsinki: Finnish Literature Society. http://scripta.kotus.fi/visk.

Hammell, K. R. (2014). Belonging, occupation, and human well-being: An exploration. *Canadian Journal of Occupational Therapy, 81*(1), 39–50.

Harra, T. (2014). *Terapeuttinen yhteistoiminta: Asiakkaan osallistumisen mahdollistaminen toimintaterapiassa* [Therapeutic collaboration: Enabling client participation in occupational therapy]. Rovaniemi: Acta Universitatis Lapponiensis.

Heritage, J. (2011). Conversation analysis: Practices and methods. In D. Silverman (Ed.), *Qualitative research: Theory, method and practice* (pp. 208–230). London: Sage.

Hibbard, J. H., & Greene, J. (2013). What the evidence shows about patient activation: Better health outcomes and care experiences; fewer data on costs. *Health Affairs, 32*(2), 207–214.

Honkasalo, M. (2013). Katveessa. Pieni toimijuus kriittisenä avauksena toiminnan teoriaan [In shades. Small agency as a critical opening to the activity theory]. *Tiede & Edistys, 1*, 42–61.

Kielhofner, G. (2002). *A model of human occupation. Theory and application.* Baltimore: Williams & Wilkins.

Parsons, T. (1937). *The structure of social action.* New York: The Free Press.

Sidnell, J., & Stivers, T. (Eds.). (2013). *The handbook of conversation analysis.* Chichester, UK: Wiley-Blackwell.

Stevanovic, M. (2012). Establishing joint decisions in a dyad. *Discourse Studies, 14*(6), 779–803.

Sumsion, T. (2006). Overview of client-centred practice. In T. Sumsion (Ed.), *Client-centred practice in occupational therapy: A guide to implementation* (pp. 1–19). Philadelphia: Elsevier.

Taylor, R. (2008). *The intentional relationship. Occupational therapy and use of self.* Philadelphia: Davis.

Weiste, E. (2018). Relational interaction in occupational therapy: Conversation analysis of positive feedback. *Scandinavian Journal of Occupational Therapy, 25*(1), 44–51.

Weiste, E., Voutilainen, L., & Peräkylä, A. (2016). Epistemic asymmetries in psychotherapy interaction: Therapists' practices for displaying access to clients' inner experiences. *Sociology of Health & Illness, 38*(4), 645–661.

WFOT. (2012). *Definition of occupational therapy.* www.wfot.org.

WHO. (2010). *User empowerment in mental health—A statement by the WHO Regional Office for Europe.* http://www.euro.who.int/__data/assets/pdf_file/0020/113834/E93430.pdf.

11

Affective Processes of Joint Meaning-Making in Couple Therapy

Evrinomy Avdi and Vasileia Lerou

Joint Decision-Making and Couple Psychotherapy

Over recent decades, the notion of shared decision-making has gained increasing popularity in healthcare provision. Within the field of mental health, actively engaging clients in decisions about their care is advocated in terms of both its clinical utility and on ethical grounds (Slade, 2017). In this chapter, we explore joint meaning-making as a specific type of joint decision-making, taking place in couple therapy. We illuminate the verbal and affective interactional processes that underlie the joint creation of meaning, which we argue is an important and often implicitly actualized aspect of the therapeutic process.

Over the least 20 years, and influenced by social constructionism, the literature on couple and family therapy approaches human systems as linguistic systems that are organized by characteristic communicative

E. Avdi (✉) · V. Lerou
Aristotle University of Thessaloniki, Thessaloniki, Greece
e-mail: avdie@psy.auth.gr

C. Lindholm et al. (eds.), *Joint Decision Making in Mental Health*,
The Language of Mental Health, https://doi.org/10.1007/978-3-030-43531-8_11

markers (Anderson & Goolishian, 1988). Accordingly, psychological problems are conceptualized as created, maintained, and dissolved in and through language and social interaction. In this framework, psychotherapy is approached as a semantic process, which entails the reconstruction of meanings (especially meanings about the problem) and the reformulation of the clients' subjectivity, reflected in changes in self-narratives and in subject positioning. A key aim of psychotherapy talk is for clients to reconstruct their life narratives in ways that are increasingly complex, emotionally salient, inclusive of experience, polyphonic and flexible (Avdi & Georgaca, 2007).

Within this framework, *problem constructions* are considered to be key to the practice of psychotherapy; through therapy talk, clients' concerns are recast into the language of therapy and thus rendered understandable within the therapy discourse and treatable through its practices. Problem constructions are not neutral as they entail issues of accountability, blame, as well as positioning and ideology (Avdi, 2015). Problem constructions implicate a cause, ascribe responsibility and imply solutions (Buttny, 2004), and as such, are relevant to processes of decision-making. Furthermore, negotiations around problem constructions are an ongoing process in psychotherapy, as clients and therapists attempt to create a joint understanding of the clients' difficulties and ways to address these.

In couple therapy, more specifically, problem constructions often involve negotiations around clienthood, that is discussions about who has the problem and who should change; these discussions are often affectively charged, and problem constructions are often contested in couple therapy (Wahlström, 2012). Partners may disagree about the causes, nature, and solutions to their difficulties; moreover, blame is a common dynamic in many distressed couples that seek help. On the other hand, couples may share a way of making sense of their difficulties, but this may be implicated in pathologizing or limiting one or both partners' well-being. As such, examining the processes through which couple therapists navigate through the complex, and often affectively charged, processes of negotiating shared meanings about the couple's distress can contribute to a better understanding of the process of couple therapy.

The Joint Creation of Meaning and Therapeutic Interaction

Several authors have argued that the establishment of a respectful and responsive conversational context, in which clients can begin to reconstruct their life narratives, is crucial for the process of therapy (Avdi & Georgaca, 2019; Smoliak & Strong, 2019). In this sense, therapy depends on the creation of "dialogical space" (Rober, 2005), which allows emotional expression, the generation of not-yet said meanings, the articulation of voices that have hitherto been silenced or excluded, and the re-organization of the clients' position repertoire (Anderson, 2012; Seikkula, 2011).

Within contemporary collaborative and dialogical approaches to couple therapy, the therapist's receptive and responsive attitude toward the clients' storytelling is considered to be a key therapeutic task that is crucial for the reconstruction of the clients' problem. Several related notions have been articulated to describe the therapists' attitude, such as adopting a "not knowing" stance (Anderson & Goolishian, 1988), participating in dialogue (Seikkula, 2011), exhibiting tolerance of uncertainty (Seikkula & Olson, 2003) and being relationally responsive (Anderson, 2012). These concepts have been debated on both theoretical and practical grounds (e.g., Guilfoyle, 2003) but they remain key principles in couple therapy practice.

In line with this, there is strong evidence that aspects of the therapeutic interactions that are associated with responsive action on the part of the therapist are crucial for the outcome of psychotherapy (Norcross, 2011). A key concept relevant to conceptualizing responsiveness and collaboration in the client-therapist relationship is the *therapeutic alliance*. The therapeutic alliance is a pan-theoretical concept that reflects the collaborative aspects of the therapeutic relationship and is seen to consist of (a) a strong emotional bond characterized by trust and (b) agreement and collaboration on the goals and the tasks of therapy (Bordin, 1979). There is strong evidence that the quality of the therapeutic alliance is predictive of outcomes in both individual and family therapy (Friedlander, Escudero, & Heatherington, 2006; Horvarth & Bedi, 2002). Similarly, in the field of shared decision-making in mental health, the establishment of a strong alliance has been described by both professionals and service users as fundamental for its implementation (Eliacin, Salyers, Kukla, & Matthias, 2015). In conjoint treatments, several competing factors affect the formation of the alliance (e.g., power dynamics and conflict in the couple, trust, loyalty, and secrets) and these render its establishment difficult (Friedlander, Escudero, Heatherington, & Diamond, 2011). In couple therapy, the alliance comprises of a web of closely interlinked, complex relationships between participants and the various subsystems thus formed (Horvarth, del Re, Flückiger, & Symonds, 2011).

Recent research has addressed in detail the interactional processes through which the therapeutic alliance is formed, maintained, challenged, and restored within sessions (Safran & Muran, 2000). Conversation-analytic research has examined aspects of the alliance in terms of alignment and affiliation. Collaboration with regard to the goals and tasks of therapy has been studied through the notion of alignment, which entails cooperative actions that facilitate a conversational sequence or activity, such as accepting and following the sequence of conversation and joint meaning-making (Muntigl & Horvarth, 2016; Sutherland & Strong, 2011). Affiliation, that is, actions that display agreement, sharedness, solidarity, understanding, and empathy (Lindstrom & Sorjonen, 2013), has been associated with the emotional bond aspect of the alliance. A key aspect of affiliation entails the listener joining in the other's emotional stance and, as such, is associated with concepts such as empathic attunement, rapport, reciprocity, engagement, and interpersonal sensitivity. In conversation, affiliation is actualized through both verbal and nonverbal means, such as continuers or minimal responses (e.g., "uh huh," "yeah," "yes") (Fitzgerald, & Leudar, 2010), repairs (Mondada, 2011), smiling, head nods (Stivers, 2008), prosody (Kykyri et al., 2017; Weiste & Peräkylä, 2014), as well as affiliative facial expressions (Chovil, 1991; Peräkylä & Ruusuvuori, 2012). In psychotherapy process research, attending to the role of nonverbal displays is arguably crucial, given that therapy entails affectively charged processes of personal narration, problem construction and identity work.

Research Questions

In this chapter, we explore the interactional processes that underlie the joint creation of new meanings, between all participants, in the context of a systemic couple therapy. We use one interactive event from a couple therapy session to examine the following research questions:

- How is the problem jointly (re)constructed in couple therapy?
- How does the therapist affectively respond to the clients' narratives in order to facilitate a joint understanding of their difficulties?

Data and Method

The research material used in this chapter was drawn from one session of couple therapy, conducted in a Family Therapy Department in Greece in the context of a wider research project (Avdi & Seikkula, 2019; Seikkula, Karvonen, Kykyri, Kaartinen, & Penttonen, 2015). The service provides couple and family therapy to the community; treatment follows systemic principles with the added use of reflective conversations (Andersen, 1987). In practice, sessions take place every three to four weeks between a primary therapist and the couple. A second therapist watches the session behind a one-way mirror and joins a conversation toward the end of each session. For the purposes of the research project, all sessions were video-recorded with four cameras, in split-screen mode. Following a naturalistic design, no changes were made in the way therapy was practiced. Couples were informed about the study by a graduate researcher and participated on a voluntary basis. Ethical approval was granted by the Family Therapy Department's Scientific Board.

Two experienced, female systemic family therapists in their fifties participated in the therapy discussed in this chapter. The therapy concerned Costas and Demetra, a white heterosexual couple in their mid-thirties. The therapy consisted of 15 sessions, spanning 14 months. The couple came to therapy because of increasing tension in their relationship, following the birth of their baby 10 months earlier. At the end of treatment, the couple reported improvement both in their personal lives and their relationship.

The research material used in this chapter consists of the video and transcript of the third session. We decided to focus on an early session, as creating a shared understanding of the problem is a key task during this stage of therapy. Furthermore, the extent of the clients' active participation in therapy is negotiated at the early stages of therapy. As such, achieving jointly constructed meanings, particularly in early sessions, is crucial for the work of therapy (Horvarth & Bedi, 2002; Knobloch-Fedders, Pinsof, & Mann, 2005).

This session was selected for analysis as it was shown to be primarily dialogical, that is to entail conversations characterized by responsiveness and mutual inquiry (Seikkula, Rober, & Laitila, 2012). The session was transcribed verbatim, following conventional conversation-analytic transcription notation, including key nonverbal displays. However, due to the nature of the analysis, which necessitates longer stretches of talk, speakers' turns, rather than lines, are numbered sequentially. Nonverbal displays of affiliation are marked in the transcript, following the respective turns. The extracts were examined using discourse analysis (Georgaca & Avdi, 2011) informed by conversation-analytic tools.

More specifically, in terms of discourse use the primary focus of the analysis was on problem constructions and their development through the session. Furthermore, we examined the speakers' responsiveness to each other's meanings with a focus on affect mirroring and displays of affiliation and empathy, as well as nonverbal displays of tension. These different modes of interaction were combined to provide a detailed description of the process of joint meaning-making in the session.

Affective and Semantic Aspects of Joint Meaning-Making in Couple Therapy

The session discussed in this chapter is used to illustrate a therapeutic conversation in which the problem is gradually jointly reconstructed, as the couple begin to elaborate on painful and delicate issues in their relationship. The therapist's stance is characterized by responsiveness to meanings that are yet not fully articulated and by affect mirroring. This way of working was typical in this therapy as a whole, and the extract analyzed illustrates several of the ways in which the therapist contributes to the creation of new meanings. Although the specifics of the meanings created are particular to this couple, the process of joint meaning-making described is arguably a key process in couple therapy. In line with dialogical principles, joint meaning-making has been shown to rely primarily on processes that elicit *narrative elaboration*, whereby not-yet articulated experiences come to be narrated and gradually assimilated into the clients' self-narratives, and processes that promote *emotional expression*.

Before turning to the extract, we outline the main problem constructions in this couple therapy and the way they develop through time. At the start of therapy, the clients construct the problem in terms of disagreements over sharing household responsibilities: Costas is not sufficiently engaged in their household, which Demetra finds frustrating. This issue is quickly resolved and the difficulties that Demetra experiences in her role as mother become the primary focus of several sessions. In this session, the narrative of the couple's difficulties gradually expands and Demetra begins to describe how she has felt depressed, trapped, and bored with her life, since the birth of their baby. She describes her baby as a "parasite" that makes constant demands on her, and reports having frequent bursts of anger, often aimed at her baby, which are followed by intense guilt. These issues are painful, delicate, and implicate troubled positioning with respect to motherhood. In the analysis that follows, we have illustrated how the delicate issue of Demetra's sadness and hopelessness is gradually introduced into the conversation, thus contributing to joint construction of new meanings for the couple's difficult experiences. We argue that the therapist's responsive stance facilitates the narration for experiences that are as yet unstoried.

The extract discussed is from the beginning of the third session, where Demetra's sadness and sense of feeling trapped is first brought into the conversation. The session starts with the couple reporting improvement; Costas is more engaged in the home and tension has subsided. Demetra introduces her sense of being "bored" with her life and their relationship, a description that Costas downplays. Just before

Extract 1, Costas states that things have improved in their relationship and that if they "try a little harder, the next steps will follow." The extract starts with the therapist inviting Costas to elaborate on this.

Extract 1

01 T: Μμ, ποιο θα ήταν το δικό σου παραπέρα; (1.0) το, το καλύτερο ας πούμε παραπέρα (3.0) με την (.)Δήμητρα;
Mmm (.) what would the next steps be for you? (1.0) the best possible next steps? (3.0) with (.) Demetra
((D picks up her bottle of water, purses her lips, drinks from her bottle. C looks down))

02 (4.2)((D stops drinking, purses her lips, looks at the bottle she is holding and begins to screw the top on. C looks down))

03 C: (6.0) Ε, hhh (4.0) ποτό σε μπαρ θέλω να σε βγάλω
(6.0) Er, hhh (4.0) I want to take you out to a bar for a drink
((D looks at C and places her bottle on the table between them))

04 D: Ποτό σε μπαρ δε βγαίναμε ούτε πριν γεννηθεί ο (γιος)
We didn't go out to bar for a drink even before (son) was born
((C looks up at D))

05 C: Γι'αυτό (.) Γι'αυτό θέλω (.) [Μου'χει λείψει]
That's why, that's why I want to, [I've missed it]
((C and T smiles. D starts to play with her hair))

06 D: [Δηλαδή ήτανε μία συνήθεια] την οποία την είχαμε κόψει ούτως ή άλλως
[This was a habit] we had stopped doing anyway
((D continues to play with her hair and looks away))

07 C: (3 Εγώ είπα ότι (.) τι θέλω (.) θέλω ένα ποτό σε μπαρ
I just said that, what I want, I want a drink in a bar

08 D: °Θέλεις ένα ποτό σε μπαρ° (.) άκου να δεις, δεν μας παίρνει να πάμε για ποτό σε μπαρ (.) όσες φορές έχουμε πάει καταστραφήκαμε (.) βραχνιάσαμε
You want a drink in a bar (.) listen to me, we can't have a drink in a bar, every time we've been, it was a disaster (.) our voice got hoarse
((D continues to play with her hair. C smiles at her and plays with his hair in exactly the same way. T frowns))

09 T: Χα-χα
Heh-heh

10 D: Ξέρω'γώ βγήκαμε γκολ, τα ποτά ήτανε χάλια πιάστηκε η πλάτη μας απ'την ορθοστασία και τα σκαμπό, εε, βούιζαν τ'αυτιά μας, χα-χα, δηλαδή δεν είμαστε για μπαρ πια
We felt awful afterwards, the drinks were crap, our backs hurt from standing up and the bar stools, our ears were buzzing, heh-heh, we are not fit for bars anymore
((D stops playing with her hair and looks at C. C plays with his hair looking down))

11 C: °[Υπερβολές]°(.) Καλά θα'ρθει το Σαββατοκύριακο, θ- (.) μην αγχώνεσαι
((C looks down, playing with his hair))
°[You're exaggerating]° (.) OK the weekend will come, w- (.) don't worry

12 D: Ναι, hhhh
yes, hhhh
((D looks down))

At the start of the extract, the therapist invites Costas to elaborate on the meaning of his expression "the next steps will follow." Therapists often use the clients' personal language, joining in their "idiolect" (Holmes, 2009). This is an element of therapist responsiveness which helps create joint understanding and establish a personal relationship (Wahlström, 2019). In terms of meaning construction, preceding Extract 1, Demetra introduced her sense of feeling "bored" with their relationship, a problem description that Costas does not take up. Instead, he focuses on positive changes and downplays any reference to the couple's difficulties. Considering this, Costas' rather vague statement ("the next steps will follow") can be seen as an attempt to shift the conversation away from what seems to be a difficult issue for them. In line with this hypothesis, following the therapist's question, Demetra displays nonverbal markers of tension (turn 02) and Costas hesitates before addressing Demetra, which he does while looking at the floor (turn 03). These nonverbal displays mark the topic of the couple's relationship as delicate. Such tensions around expressing one's experience in the presence of one's intimate partner and the associated anxiety about what one's partner may choose to disclose are quite common in couple therapy (Friedlander et al., 2006), and may restrict what each client chooses to discuss. This may exclude important aspects of lived experience for one or both partners, with adverse implications for shared meaning-making.

In response to the therapist's invitation (turn 01) Costas expresses, with hesitation, his wish to take Demetra out for a drink (turn 02). A brief exchange follows, in which Demetra rejects Costas' invitation by appealing to facts with increasing emphasis (turns 04, 06, and 08). Through these turns, Demetra speaks in an increasingly assertive tone and lists in vivid detail the reasons why they cannot go to a bar (turn 08). Vivid descriptions and lists are considered to be rhetorical strategies of factualization that render an account credible and thus difficult to dispute (Edwards & Potter, 1992). On his part, Costas displays affiliation (smiles), speaks in an apologetic and conciliatory tone and appeals to his feelings (turns 05 and 07). Furthermore, during Demetra's last turn (turn 08) Costas exactly mirrors Demetra's movements. This is an example of non-conscious mimicry, a common aspect of human interaction that has been associated with affiliation and affective sharing (Chartrand & van Baaren, 2009). We could speculate that one aspect of the couple's (presumably habitual) complementary conflict style is enacted in this brief exchange: Costas makes an affiliation attempt, Demetra rejects it with irritation, Costas displays further affiliation, and so on. The therapist allows the couple's interaction to take place and observes it, while displaying several back-channel signs of attentiveness, such as smiling, gaze, and facial expression. She intervenes only when the interaction has been completed.

In sum, in Extract 1, the therapist's question invites elaboration on the couple's relationship, which is associated with tension for both partners. Following from this invitation to elaborate, difficulties in the couple's relationship are not only narrated but also displayed; this allows for deepened exploration, as will be seen in the extracts that follow.

Next, the therapist focuses on Demetra's lack of interest in the couple's joint life, thus inviting further elaboration on this difficult topic, as illustrated in Extract 2.

Extract 2

13 T: Εσύ δηλαδή, αν καταλαβαίνω, Δήμητρα, αυτό που θα'θελες
είναι να είστε οι δυο σας στο σπίτι; (1.5)
So, you, if I understand, Demetra, what you would like
is for the two of you to be at home together?
((C continues to play with his hair. D looks down and
then turns her head slowly and looks at therapist. C
looks down))

14 D: (1.5) [Δεν ξέρω]
(1.5) [I don't know]

15 C: [°Έτσι°]
[°Right°]

16 T: Άντε και με κάποιους φίλους;
with some friends at most?

17 D: °Δεν ξέρω°
°I don't know°
((D looks at the bottle in her hands))

18 T: [Έτσι που το λες]
[the way you're talking]

19 C: °[Αν μπορούσαμε να βγούμε απ' το σπίτι]°
°[if we could just go out of the house]°

20 T: λίγο βόλτα δε θες, λίγο μπαρ δε θες, λίγο(.)δεν ξέρω (.)
τι θέλεις
You don't want to go out, you don't want to go to a bar
I don't know (.) what you want
((At the end of the turn T purses her lips, lifts eyebrows
and frowns, as she displays negative affect. D looks
down))

21 (8.0)((D plays with the bottle in her hand, looks down,
makes 'shrug face', then looks at C. C sighs. D laughs.
C shakes his head and starts to drink from his bottle))

In turn 13 the therapist addresses Demetra and thus affects the course of the conversation by marking her response as relevant to the problem construction. Therapists often manage turn-taking to focus selectively on specific issues or interrupt problematic interactional patterns. In this case, the therapist addresses Demetra with a *reformulation*, which selectively focuses on specific aspects of what has been said by the previous speaker and in this way changes it, while seemingly accepting it. Reformulations are routinely used to promote therapeutic work (Antaki, 2008; Buttny, 2004; Davis, 1986; Weiste & Peräkylä, 2013). In this instance, the therapist positively reframes Demetra's rejection of Costas' invitation, as her wanting to spend time with him at home. *Positive reframing* is a key rhetorical practice in family therapy and an alliance-building strategy (Friedlander et al., 2006). She introduces this reformulation tentatively, with a hedge expression ("if I understand"), thus inviting collaboration. Over the next couple of turns, the therapist builds on her reformulation (turn 16) while Demetra resists it, by repeating "I don't know" (turns 14 and 17). Demetra does not express her disagreement directly but rather withdraws from the conversation, a non-preferred response in therapy talk. Clients' minimal responses to the therapists' interventions are considered to be markers of withdrawal ruptures (Eubanks, Muran, & Safran, 2015) that reflect troubled collaboration.

Next, the therapist changes track and challenges Demetra's lack of response more directly (turns 18 and 20); her intervention concludes with "I don't know what you want." With this latter statement, the therapist shifts the focus of conversation to the here-and-now, using Demetra's own words again. This is an example of metacommunication, one of the strategies therapists use to repair alliance ruptures (Eubanks et al., 2015). Through this intervention, the therapist illuminates the troubled collaboration between herself and Demetra and renders it relevant to their conversation. Importantly, there is a marked change toward negative affect in the therapist's facial expression in turn 20, as she reflects in an exaggerated manner Demetra's affective state. Successful affect mirroring has been shown to consist of affective displays that are contingent on the original expression but marked; that is, different in intensity (Holmes, 2009). Therapists often exaggerate the affective display of clients, thus encouraging the expression of emotion with increased salience and depth. During this exchange, Costas joins in, in a quiet voice that overlaps with the therapist's turns (turns 15 and 19) but does not interrupt them, and in fact aligns with them.

However, the therapist's attempt to repair the alliance with Demetra and explore her experience is met with further resistance, as she withdraws further: Demetra does not respond to the therapist's invitation, makes a "shrug face," turns to Costas and laughs in a conspiratorial manner (turn 21), presumably in an attempt to shift focus. Costas displays signs of both tension and affiliation (turn 21), before taking the floor and introducing a new issue, as discussed in Extract 3.

The above exchange is quite complex with respect to the therapy process; the therapist works at maintaining an alliance with both partners through different modalities of communication. On a semantic level, the therapist's turns (13, 16, 18, and 20) align with Costas' account that the problem is associated with Demetra's lack of interest. At the same time, the therapist affiliates with Demetra on a nonverbal level, through mirroring her affect and on a verbal level through addressing the difficulties in their current interaction (turn 20). In this way, the therapist maintains the therapeutic alliance with Costas (as she aligns with his problem description) and at the same time, attempts to repair the alliance with Demetra (through metacommunication and affect mirroring). In other words, the therapist *joins in* with both partners through different modalities.

The interaction that follows (Extract 3) is important in terms of joint meaning-making. Costas introduces a difficult topic for the couple, their sex life, and the interaction culminates in the expression of strong affect. The problem construction expands and becomes more inclusive of lived experience, strong emotions are expressed, and thus aspects of the couple's experience that had been hitherto excluded, enter the conversation.

Extract 3

22 C: Το σεξ περνάει απ' το μυαλό σου καθόλου;
Does sex cross your mind at all?
((C takes a sip from his drink, looks at D, puts his bottle down and crosses his arms))

23 T: Αχά!
Aha!
((T puts her glasses on and smiles))

24 D: Δεν θέλω να κάνω σεξ(.)βαριέμαι
I don't want to have sex (.) I am bored
((D takes bottle to her mouth and drinks))

25 C: Ανά σαράντα μέρες, πενήντα (.)
Every forty days, fifty

26 D: χα-χα
heh-heh

27 C: Ο ήλιος (.) το φεγγάρι που κάθε πρωί-
the sun (.) the moon that every morning-
((C speaks in a light-hearted tone. D stops drinking and wipes her mouth. T smiles))

28 D: Αφού βαριέμαι ρε [παιδί μου]
but I am bored
((D's facial expression changes to negative affect, she leans forward, puts bottle on table))

29 C: Ναι(.) το κατ-, το αντιλαμβάνομαι αυτό
Yes (.) I under- I am aware of that
((C speaks in a gentle voice, smiling))

30 D: Μου είναι τρομερά:: δύσκολη διαδικασία (.) δεν μπορώ (.) Κουράζομαι
It is a terribly:: difficult process for me (.) I can't (.) I feel tired

31 ((D picks up a tissue from the table and sits back again. T frowns and looks at D with concern. D takes her glasses off, she looks sad. C looks at her smiling. D starts to cry))

32 T: ↓Κουράζεσαι?
You feel tired?

33 (21.0) ((D puts the tissue over her eyes and cries. C looks at her with a frozen smile, the smile gradually fades and he then bites his lip. D continues to cry, T looks at D with an expression of empathic concern. Eventually, D puts the tissue down, puts her glasses on, sighs and looks down))

34 C: Δεν σε πιέζω προς κάποια κατεύθυνση (3.0) αλήθεια το λέω
I am not putting pressure on you (3.0) I mean it
((C smiles at D; D looks down and sighs))

35 (5.0)((C picks up his bottle of water and opens it.
D looks down, sniffs))

36 D: <Tι να πω• Δεν δέοω τι να πω> (1.5)
<What can I say? I don't know what to say> (1.5)

37 T: ↓Θες να κλάψεις?
You want to cry?

38 (11.0)((D cries. C plays with the bottle in his hands,
looks at D briefly, then leans forward and looks down))

39 D: Συγνώμη (10.0) δεν ξέρω τι θα μπορούσαμε να κάνουμε (.)
ειλικρινά
I am sorry (10.0) I don't know what we could do (.)
honestly

At the start of the extract, Costas takes the initiative to introduce another delicate issue, the couple's sexual relationship (turn 22). It seems that the therapist's responsiveness in the previous turn contributed to the establishment of safety, which in turn facilitated this difficult conversation to take place. The therapist marks this as important with an emphatic continuer (turn 23). In response, Demetra states that she is "bored" with sex and displays signs of tension (turn 24); boredom is a rather vague emotion, often used to disguise more intense negative affect. Costas persists in talking about sex, in a light-hearted, humorous way (turns 25 and 27) and initially Demetra joins in his light tone and laughs (turn 26). However, her expression soon shifts to negative affect as she repeats, more emphatically, that she is bored (turn 28). Costas, presumably sensitive to Demetra's distress, quickly aligns with her, affirming that he understands her feelings and smiles (turn 29). This responsive move on Costas' part facilitates emotional expression and Demetra begins to talk about how difficult she finds sex and how tired she feels (turn 30). In terms of problem construction, this is an important development; the initially rather vague affective state of being bored becomes one of struggling, finding things difficult and feeling tired. Similarly, in terms of affect, diffuse tension is replaced by the expression of sadness. These shifts reflect a process whereby the couple's narratives about their difficulties become richer, more inclusive, and emotionally salient, in line with the aims of psychotherapy.

In terms of meaning-making, it is interesting to note the differing responses by Costas and the therapist to Demetra crying. Faced with Demetra's tears Costas smiles, presumably in an effort to cheer her up. On the other hand, the therapist's facial expression changes drastically from smiling to negative affect, mirroring Demetra's sadness (turn 31), and then she asks gently, in a soft, soothing voice, repeating Demetra's exact wording "you feel tired?" (turn 32). The use of soft prosody and low vocal tone is a conversational tool that conveys affiliation and affect attunement that can promote the process of change in therapy (Kykyri et al., 2017; Weiste & Peräkylä, 2014). Furthermore, from a clinical perspective, turn 33 illustrates therapeutic change on a nonverbal level, as the therapist's responsive focus on Demetra's feelings of sadness (turn 32) disrupts a presumably habitual interactional pattern in the couple, which functions to exclude sadness from being expressed. Interestingly, Costas' facial expression also changes to negative affect, following the therapist's intervention. When Demetra's crying subsides (end of turn 33), Costas makes another affiliative opening (turn 34) but Demetra withdraws (turn 35). Instead, the therapist focuses on Demetra's affective experience (turn 36); she says, "you want to cry," in a low quiet voice and a sad facial expression, an invitation that deepens Demetra's affective expression. Following this interaction, and when her crying eventually subsides, Demetra begins to express her sadness, helplessness, and sense of despair (turn 38), topics which are further elaborated on in the remaining session.

In sum, in the interaction described above, the couple's problem construction expands to include Demetra's affectively charged struggles with motherhood, her depression and sense of helplessness, as well as Costas' frustration and guilt in managing these strong feelings. The therapist contributes to these shifts primarily through empathic responsiveness and affect mirroring. The interaction described is an example of a process of joint meaning-making, whereby painful experiences for the couple begin to be expressed and a dialogical space is created in which new meanings regarding the couple's life can gradually develop.

Conclusions

In this chapter, we illustrated some of the interactional processes involved in joint meaning-making in the context of couple therapy. We presented in detail an interactive event, which illustrates the therapist's agenda and practices of promoting emotional expression and joint narrative elaboration of delicate issues in the couple's life. Although our analysis focused on only one brief interactive episode, we propose that circumscribed events can activate processes of dramatic change, in line with the tenets of dynamic systems theory (Salvatore, Tschacher, Gelo, & Koch, 2015).

In line with the principles of collaborative and dialogical approaches to couple therapy, a key aim of therapy is to create a dialogical space that allows the narration of aspects of experience that are as yet unstoried, and thus to facilitate the expansion and reconstruction of the couple's difficulties and self-narratives. Analysis of the session as a whole and as illustrated in the extracts presented, highlighted the therapist's affective responsiveness to the clients' storytelling as key aspects of this process. The therapist's verbal interventions were minimal, as she used primarily continuers, repairs (often repeating the clients' exact words) and, less frequently, reformulations. In other words, most of the therapist's utterances were oriented toward establishing intersubjective understanding rather than directly shifting meaning. Although subtle, these interventions powerfully affected the unfolding conversation toward the creation of new, shared meanings. In other words, the therapist was active in creating the conditions for dialogue and jointly created meanings, primarily through responsiveness and affect mirroring. As a result, difficult feelings began to be expressed and the clients' narratives became richer, more complex and more emotionally salient.

Previous discursive research has highlighted the more active rhetorical strategies that family therapists use to challenge, deconstruct, expand, and reverse problem-saturated accounts and to promote positive, solution-focused and relational descriptions of the family's difficulties (e.g., Avdi & Georgaca, 2007; Smoliak & Strong, 2019). There is evidence that therapists use strategies such as direct questions, information-eliciting tellings and reformulations to elicit client narration (Buttny, 2004; Davis, 1986). In this case, however, the primary way in which the therapist contributed to narrative elaboration was through affiliation and affective responsiveness. This finding complements previous research and highlights the importance of studying nonverbal displays alongside language use when studying psychotherapy process.

This study focused on a good outcome case and a session characterized by collaboration; it would be interesting to extend this inquiry by studying so-called "monological" clinical interventions, i.e., conversations during which joint meaning-making is compromised, in order to deepen our understanding of the challenges implicated in this endeavor and to explore possible solutions to these.

The findings of this small-scale study have implications for psychotherapy theory, practice and research. More specifically, the findings highlight the importance for the therapy process of establishing a shared semantic framework, promoting collaboration, and establishing a therapeutic alliance. Moreover, the importance of a relationally responsive stance on the part of the therapist for fostering the creation of a healing conversation is underscored. Furthermore, the analysis illustrates that joint meaning-making in therapy is not always given, as clients often "resist" invitation to explore difficult feelings and experiences. Therapists need to work actively toward establishing alliance and collaboration and to creating conditions of safety where clients can risk exploring painful experiences.

References

Andersen, T. (1987). The reflecting team: Dialogue and meta-dialogue in clinical work. *Family Process, 26*(4), 415–428.

Anderson, H. (2012). Collaborative relationships and dialogical conversations: Ideas for a relationally responsive practice. *Family Process, 51*(1), 8–24.

Anderson, H., & Goolishian, H. (1988). Human systems as linguistic systems: Preliminary and evolving ideas about the implications for clinical theory. *Family Process, 27*(4), 371–393.

Antaki, C. (2008). Formulations in psychotherapy. In A. Peräkylä, C. Antaki, S. Vehviläinen, & I. Leudar (Eds.), *Conversation analysis and psychotherapy* (pp. 26–42). Cambridge: Cambridge University Press.

Avdi, E. (2015). Fostering dialogue: Exploring the therapists' discursive contributions in a couple therapy. In M. Borcsa & P. Rober (Eds.), *Research perspectives in couple therapy: Discursive qualitative methods* (pp. 71–88). Heidelberg: Springer.

Avdi, E., & Georgaca, E. (2007). Discourse analysis and psychotherapy: A critical review. *European Journal of Psychotherapy and Counselling, 9*(2), 157–176.

Avdi, E., & Georgaca, E. (2019). Researching the discursive construction of subjectivity in psychotherapy. In O. Smoliak & T. Strong (Eds.), *Therapy as discourse: Practice and research* (pp. 45–70). London: Palgrave.

Avdi, E., & Seikkula, J. (2019). Studying the process of psychoanalytic psychotherapy: Discursive and embodied aspects. *British Journal of Psychotherapy, 35*(2), 217–232.

Bordin, E. S. (1979). The generalizability of the psychoanalytic concept of the working alliance. *Psychotherapy: Theory, Research & Practice, 16*(3), 252–260.

Buttny, R. (2004). *Talking problems: Studies on discursive construction*. Albany: State University of New York Press.

Chartrand, T. L., & van Baaren, R. (2009). Human mimicry. In M. P. Zanna (Ed.), *Advances in experimental social psychology* (pp. 219–274). Cambridge: Elsevier.

Chovil, N. (1991). Discourse-oriented facial displays in conversation. *Research on Language and Social Interaction, 25,* 163–194.

Davis, K. (1986). The process of problem (re)formulation in psychotherapy. *Sociology of Health & Illness, 8*(1), 44–74.

Edwards, D., & Potter, J. (1992). *Discursive psychology*. London: Sage.

Eliacin, J., Salyers, M. P., Kukla, M., & Matthias, M. S. (2015). Patients' understanding of shared decision making in a mental health setting. *Qualitative Health Research, 25*(5), 668–678.

Eubanks, C. F., Muran, J. C., & Safran, J. D. (2015). *Rupture resolution rating system (3RS): Manual.* Unpublished manuscript. New York: Mount Sinai-Beth Israel Medical Centre.

Fitzgerald, P., & Leudar, I. (2010). On active listening in person-centred, solution-focused psychotherapy. *Journal of Pragmatics, 42*(12), 3188–3198.

Friedlander, M. L., Escudero, V., & Heatherington, L. (2006). *Therapeutic alliances in couple and family therapy: An empirically informed guide to practice*. Washington, DC: American Psychological Association.

Friedlander, M. L., Escudero, V., Heatherington, L., & Diamond, G. M. (2011). Alliance in couple and family therapy. *Psychotherapy, 48*(1), 25–33.

Georgaca, E., & Avdi, E. (2011). Discourse analysis. In D. J. Harper & A. Thompson (Eds.), *Qualitative research methods in mental health and psychotherapy: An introduction for students and practitioners* (pp. 147–162). Chichester, UK: Wiley.

Guilfoyle, M. (2003). Dialogue and power: A critical analysis of power in family therapy. *Family Process, 42*(3), 331–343.

Holmes, J. (2009). *Exploring in security: Towards an attachment-informed psychoanalytic psychotherapy*. London: Routledge.

Horvarth, A. O., Del Re, A., Flückiger, C., & Symonds, D. (2011). Alliance in individual therapy. *Psychotherapy, 48*(1), 9–16.

Horvath, A. O., & Bedi, R. P. (2002). The alliance. In J. C. Norcross (Ed.), *Psychotherapy relationships that work: Therapist contributions and responsiveness to patients* (pp. 37–69). Oxford: Oxford University Press.

Knobloch-Fedders, L., Pinsof, W. M., & Mann, B. J. (2005). The formation of the therapeutic alliance in couple therapy. *Family Process, 43*(4), 425–442.

Kykyri, V. L., Tourunen, A., Wahlström, J., Kaartinen, J., Penttonen, M., & Seikkula, J. (2017). Soft prosody and embodied attunement in therapeutic interaction: A multimethod case study of a moment of change. *Journal of Constructivist Psychology, 30*(3), 211–234.

Lindstrom, A., & Sorjonen, M.-L. (2013). Affiliation in conversation. In J. Sidnell & T. Stivers (Eds.), *The handbook of conversation analysis* (pp. 350–369). London: Wiley.

Mondada, L. (2011). Understanding as an embodied, situated and sequential achievement in interaction. *Journal of Pragmatics, 43*(2), 542–552.

Muntigl, P., & Horvarth, A. (2016). A conversation analytic study of building and repairing the alliance in family therapy. *Journal of Family Therapy, 38*(1), 102–119.

Norcross, J. C. (2011). Evidence-based therapy relationships: Research conclusions and clinical practices. *Psychotherapy Theory, Research, Practice Training, 48*(1), 98–102.

Peräkylä, A., & Ruusuvuori, J. (2012). Facial expression in an assessment. In H. Knoblauch, B. Schentter, & J. Raab (Eds.), *Video analysis: Methodology and methods* (pp. 127–142). Oxford: Peter Lang.

Rober, P. (2005). Family therapy as a dialogue of living persons. *Journal of Marital and Family Therapy, 31*(4), 385–397.

Safran, J. D., & Muran, J. C. (2000). *Negotiating the therapeutic alliance: A relational treatment guide*. London: Guilford.

Salvatore, S., Tschacher, W., Gelo, O. C. G., & Koch, S. C. (2015). Dynamic systems theory and embodiment in psychotherapy research: A new look at process and outcome. *Frontiers in Psychology, 6,* 914.

Seikkula, J. (2011). Becoming dialogical: Psychotherapy or a way of life? *Australian & New Zealand Journal of Family Therapy, 32*(3), 179–193.

Seikkula, J., Karvonen, A., Kykyri, V.-L., Kaartinen, J., & Penttonen, M. (2015). The embodied attunement of therapists and a couple within dialogical psychotherapy: An introduction to the relational mind project. *Family Process, 54*(4), 703–715.

Seikkula, J., & Olson, M. (2003). The open dialogue approach to acute psychosis: Its poetics and micropolitics. *Family Process, 42*(3), 403–418.

Seikkula, J., Rober, P., & Laitila, A. (2012). Making sense of multi-actor dialogues in family therapy and network meetings. *Journal of Marital and Family Therapy, 38*(4), 667–687.

Slade, M. (2017). Implementing shared decision making in routine mental health care. *World Psychiatry, 16*(2), 146–153.

Smoliak, O., & Strong, T. (Eds.). (2019). *Therapy as discourse: Practice and research*. London: Palgrave.

Stivers, T. (2008). Stance, alignment, and affiliation during storytelling: When nodding is a token of affiliation. *Research on Language and Social Interaction, 41*(1), 31–57.

Sutherland, O., & Strong, T. (2011). Therapeutic collaboration: A conversation analysis of constructionist therapy. *Journal of Family Therapy, 33*(3), 256–278.

Wahlström, J. (2012). Constructing the moral order of a relationship in couples therapy. In M. Borcsa & P. Rober (Eds.), *Research perspectives in couple therapy: Discursive qualitative methods* (pp. 149–166). Heidelberg: Springer.

Wahlström, J. (2019). Discourse in psychotherapy: Using words to create therapeutic practice. In O. Smoliak & T. Strong (Eds.), *Therapy as discourse: Practice and research* (pp. 19–44). London: Palgrave.

Weiste, E., & Peräkylä, A. (2013). A comparative conversation analytic study of formulations in psychoanalysis and cognitive psychotherapy. *Research on Language and Social Interaction, 46*(4), 299–321.

Weiste, E., & Peräkylä, A. (2014). Prosody and empathic communication in psychotherapy interaction. *Psychotherapy Research, 24*(6), 687–701.

12

Standards of Interaction in Mental Health Rehabilitation: The Case of "Consensus-Based" Decisions

Taina Valkeapää, Melisa Stevanovic, Elina Weiste, and Camilla Lindholm

The Ideal of Consensus in Community-Based Rehabilitation Ideology

According to the community-based rehabilitation ideology, mental health problems are not only problems of the individual, but they are also caused by social alienation. Community membership has been found to support

---

T. Valkeapää (✉) · M. Stevanovic · E. Weiste
University of Helsinki, Helsinki, Finland
e-mail: taina.valkeapaa@helsinki.fi

M. Stevanovic
e-mail: melisa.stevanovic@helsinki.fi

E. Weiste
e-mail: elina.weiste@ttl.fi

C. Lindholm
Tampere University, Tampere, Finland
e-mail: camilla.lindholm@tuni.fi

C. Lindholm et al. (eds.), *Joint Decision Making in Mental Health*,
The Language of Mental Health, https://doi.org/10.1007/978-3-030-43531-8_12

the relationships of mental health clients with other people and to enhance their well-being (Lawson, 2016). Communities seek to increase individuals' engagement and responsibility through joint activities. Since responsibility goes together with opportunities to influence, all decisions related to the running of the community are made together (De Leon, 2000). A consensus-based decision-making model is considered as central to the inclusion and empowerment of the individual and to the cohesion of the community (Hänninen, 2012).

The idea in community-based rehabilitation is that all clients share a common understanding of the principles that guide the activities (Haapamäki, Kaipio, Keskinen, Uusitalo, & Kuoksa, 2000). Thus, the governing principles cannot simply operate as professional practices, but require all members of the community to be *socialized into* them (Kaipio, 1999). It is argued that this socialization enables all members to have equal opportunities to act (Haapamäki et al., 2000, pp. 30–31).

Clubhouses consist of communities of clients with mental health-related problems and hired support workers. These communities are organized around a work-ordered day which is jointly planned and implemented with clients and support workers (Hänninen, 2012). It is thought that sharing responsibility for the daily life of the community brings clients closer together and thus makes the community stronger (De Leon, 2000). Membership in a community has been shown to help clients to regain their self-confidence, as well as to rediscover their social value as citizens (Tanaka, Craig, & Davidson, 2016; Tanaka & Davidson, 2015).

Membership of a Clubhouse community entails participation in joint decision-making (Hänninen, 2012). The International Quality Standards for Clubhouses state that decision-making should be based on consensus (Clubhouse International, 2019). Consensus refers to a decision-making process that not only follows the majority decision, but also takes everyone's views into account. It seems to maximize joint understanding and acceptability of the decisions. In this article, we have examined how consensus-based decisions are sought after in multi-party conversations at Clubhouse meetings.

Consensus and Communication: The Case of Habermas

Consensus is an important notion in Jürgen Habermas's (1981, 1988) analysis of modernity, liberative democracy, and communicative action. Habermas (1981, p. 107) sees modernity as a fragmented universe of different cultural spheres of value which the "lifeworld" can bring together. The lifeworld consists of cultural patterns of interpretation, evaluation, and expression shared by all actors, which provides an opportunity for mutual understanding, dialogue, and consensus-based solutions to many problems of modernity (Habermas, 1988, p. 203). The aim of language use is consensus-seeking "communicative action" (Scambler, 2001). In an "ideal speech situation," participants of equal status treat each other with respect, judging each other's assertions solely because of reason and evidence while being motivated by the common good (Habermas, 1973). They use linguistic and non-linguistic expressions in the same ways, bring all relevant arguments into the dialogue, and allow everyone to participate, express their attitudes, and introduce or question any proposal without a sense of internal or external compulsion (Jones, 2001; Walker & Lovat, 2016, p. 573).

Habermas's account has been criticized for various reasons. One point of criticism concerns his lack of adequate notice of the unequal power relations that characterize modernity (Jones, 2001, p. 175), affect individuals' differentiated access to the public sphere, and thus lead to essential "deliberative inequalities" (Bohman, 1996, p. 110). Besides overt power asymmetries, Habermas has also been seen to fail to take enough notice of "communicative inequalities" which account for individuals' differentiated capacities to make effective use of available opportunities to deliberate in the public sphere (Bohman, 1996). In other words, there are individuals who are not able to speak up and present an argument for their case, but whose presumed preferences would still "need to be imputed wherever possible" (Walker & Lovat, 2016, p. 579).

It thus appears that the only way to approach the Habermasian ideal of consensus-based decision-making in the face of the above-mentioned problems involves education: teaching of consensus-making skills and socialization participants to value that type of decision-making. In our view, such socialization practices can take three forms. First, the practices of *vicarious participation* may function as a step toward constructing the outcome of the dialogue discursively and rhetorically as consensus. Although such an outcome runs the risk of being something that Scheff (1967, p. 39) referred to as "false consensus," it may still serve to establish and reinforce the ideal of consensus as the participants' common goal. Second, the existence of consensus is subject to both *prospective and retrospective framing* (Haug, 2015), which similarly educates participants to appreciate the need for reaching consensus. Third, socialization into consensus-based decision-making may involve *explicit opposition to unilateral decision-making*—that is, against the idea of allowing a specific subset of participants to make the decisions for the whole group or community (Walker & Lovat, 2016, p. 579).

For this paper, we analyzed video-recorded data from real-life decision-making encounters in a mental health rehabilitation community, from which we cannot exclude the occurrence of deep communicative inequalities between the participants. In our analysis, we describe how the participants orient to the Habermasian ideal of consensus-based decision-making in and through their interactional practices.

Consensus-Based Decision-Making and Interaction

When does consensus emerge in interaction? The moment of consensus has been associated with synchronized nodding at the end of negotiations (Oshima, 2014), the facilitator articulating the consensus, or the last person to object to the proposal expressing an altered opinion that aligns with the opinions of the other participants (Wasson, 2016). Urfalino (2014) uses the concept *rule of non-opposition* to describe the final stage of consensus decision-making, when disagreement is absent. While participants' preferences are private knowledge that is not accessible to other participants and to the analysts, consensus can be observed by a lack of expressed disagreement.

Using Urfalino's theory as a basis, Haug (2015) describes four types of consensus decisions, which exhibit different levels of openness to disagreement. First, in *imposed consensus*, the chair announces the decision and directly moves to the next topic or closes the meeting, in which case the expression of disagreement is difficult. Second, in *acclaimed consensus*, there are explicit slots to express disagreement, but these are rarely used. Third, in *basic consensus*, participants are explicitly asked about disagreement and their silence establishes consensus. Fourth and finally, in *deliberative consensus*, participants are strongly encouraged to express their opinions. The aim is to consider disagreements openly, and to "find ways to integrate them into the "consensus-to-be" so as to make it acceptable to all" (Haug, 2015, p. 575). A relevant aspect in achieving this type of consensus is a non-restrictive atmosphere, in which each individual's opinion is respected, and the decision-making process proceeds at an unhurried pace (see Chapter 6). It is not only the shared outcome that is crucial in deliberative consensus, but also the process itself (Haug, 2015, pp. 575–576). While the participants may not totally agree with the outcome, they can let the decision stand if they think that their opinions have been heard during the discussion (Haug, 2015). This kind of consensus seems to match the ideological principles of the Clubhouse community described above.

Haug's theorizing can be complemented by Wasson's (2016) classification of the different sequence types that emerge between the proposal and the achievement of consensus. In evaluating the proposal, the participants make positive and negative assessments, which Wasson (2016, p. 388) connects to *agreement* and *disagreement*. While agreement is expressed quickly after the proposal, disagreement sequences are delayed and involve extra interactional work to bring about consensus. Wasson (2016) shows how disagreement sequences may be followed by *information sequences*, in which participants request or offer more information on the proposed activity or *joking sequences* in which laughter is employed to "repair the relationship among participants after the tension of extended disagreement" (Wasson, 2016, p. 389).

In sum, *the management of disagreement* appears to be pivotal in consensus-based decision-making: how open the discussion is to the views of all participants, including divergent opinions, and how disagreements are managed in the interaction to end up in a situation of non-opposition, consensus.

Research Questions

In this chapter, we have explored consensus-based decision-making in a mental health rehabilitation community, where these types of decisions are ideologically preferred. The research questions are:

1. How do participants display orientation to the ideal of consensus-based decision-making through interactional practices?
2. How are disagreements treated in the discussions?

Data and Method

This study is part of a larger research project on social interaction in mental health rehabilitation. The data used in the study consisted of 29 video-recorded meetings of a rehabilitation group, collected at a Finnish Clubhouse. Each meeting was attended by 2–10 clients and 1–3 support workers trained in social work. The themes dealt with during these meetings varied (see Chapters 2, 6, 8, and 10) but clients' socialization into the practices of consensus-based decision-making was an important part of all this. The participants gave their informed consent for the data collection. Approval of the research ethics was obtained from the Southern Finland Clubhouse Association (date of the decision: 19.09.2016), and research permission was issued by the Board of Directors at the Clubhouses in the relevant area.

The method used in the study was conversation analysis (Schegloff, 2007; Sidnell & Stivers, 2013). Conversation analysis seeks to unravel reoccurring interactional practices through which social actions are constructed in moment-by-moment processes—something that may be seen to represent an instance of "sociological miniaturism" (Stolte, Fine, & Cook, 2001). In our analysis, we focused on the turn-by-turn unfolding of joint decision-making sequences. First, we engaged in qualitative case-by-case analysis of a wider collection of joint decision-making sequences ($N=455$), identified in our data set. Then, we focused more specifically on the sequences where the participants' orientations to consensus became visible at the surface level of interaction. The data extracts presented below were based on their capacity to demonstrate the variety of these participant orientations.

Analysis: The Notion of Consensus as a Local Resource

We organize our analysis of how consensus-based decision-making becomes visible in the Clubhouse support workers' interactional practices in the following way. First, we consider how decision-making can be prospectively framed as consensus-based. Second, we describe how consensus is aimed at disagreements and how they are treated during the decision-making processes. Third, we illustrate how the decision-making process is framed retrospectively to match with the ideals of consensus-based decision-making.

The Prospective Framing of Interaction

Decision-making processes are sometimes preceded by framing the current circumstances prospectively as favorable for consensus-based decision-making. This is the case in Extract 1, where a support worker (SW1) outlines why the situation is opportune for deciding a procedure on how to select an employee for the Clubhouse's "transitional employment" program.

Extract 1

01 SW1: mutta, (.) käviskö nyt sillä tavalla että tehtäs
but (.) would it now be ok if we would

02 tänää nyt yhdessä pohditaan koska nyt on hyvä (0.4)
today now discuss together 'cause now there's (0.4)

03 määrä ihmisiä tässä. (.) niin me voidaan niinkun,
a good number of people here (.) so we can like,

04 (1.0) ihan hyvillä mielin tehdä tää
(1.0) in quite good spirits do this

05 siirtymätyöntekijän valinta, (.) prosessinkuvaus
process description of choosing transitional employee

06 tähän et miten me halutaan koska täs on nyt niinku,
here what we want because here we now have

07 (1.0) ehkä se tärkein porukkakin jotka on
(1.0) perhaps the key people who are

08 kiinnostuneita siihen työhön lähtemiseen ja,
interested in starting work and,

09 (0.2) näin niin, (1.4) ni tulee sit semmone, (1.6)
(0.2) so well, (1.4) then we have that, (1.6)

10 sellaset, (.) sellanen niinku, (1.4) valinta, (0.2)
that kind, (.) that kind of, (1.4) choice, (0.2)

11 systeemi tohon kirjotettua et kaikki
system written there so everybody

12 ollaan tyytyväisiä.
is satisfied

((5 lines omitted: Esa asks if the work is part-time))

```
13       (2.0)

14 SW1: mut käviskö se et tehään nyt tää, (.) tää kuvaus.
        would it be okay if we now (.) do this description

15      (0.4) sit meil on niinku yks asia, (.) selkee, (0.4)
        (0.4) then we have like one thing, (.) clear, (0.4)

16      sit voidaan kattoo tätä, (0.8) ryhmäaikatauluu.
        then we can look at this (0.8) group schedule

17 SW2: °mm° ((nyökkäilee))
         mm ((nods))

18      (3.0)

19 SW1: ja sit jos jää viel aikaa ni voidaan rupatella
        and then if we still have time we can talk about

20      mistä halutaan.
        whatever we want

21 Esa: no ni alotetaan sitte.
        okay let's start

22      (3.0)

23 SW1: käykö.
        is it okay

24 Maj: joo.
        yeah

25 Kia: käy.
        it's okay
26 Aki: jo.
        yes
```

Extract 1 is from the beginning of the meeting. SW1 describes the circumstances at the meeting as optimal for deciding about the employee selection procedure: there is a good number of people present (lines 2–3) and these are the very people who will be affected by the decision (lines 7–8). Thus, SW1 addresses those local and situational elements in the current social and physical context that are adequate for a consensus-based decision. SW1 also stresses the need to reach a decision that everybody finds acceptable. First, he describes a causal relationship between the number of participants and the possibility of establishing the procedure "in good spirits" (lines 2–4). Second, he mentions the presence of the most important target group and the action of writing down a procedure that satisfies everybody (lines 7–12). Third, he repeats the proposal with reduced form in order to engage the clients in the discussion (lines 14, 23). Thus, using thorough argumentation, SW1 defines the current situation as one in which everybody can participate in the forthcoming discussion and which can lead to a decision that everybody can accept.

The support worker's prospective framing of the decision-making process appears to encourage participants to contribute to the process. This can be considered essential in the Clubhouse context, because participation in decision-making is a crucial aspect of the sense of belonging to the community, but at the same time the lack of active participation is typically a challenge to clients (see Chapter 2).

Consensus: The Management of Disagreement

Consensus decision-making is mostly about the management of disagreements: how open the discussion is to divergent opinions and whether participants can find a decision that no one opposes. Below we present two ways of arriving at non-opposition.

The following extract features a discussion in which two clients express differing opinions about the proposed activity. After a few rather reluctant responses, the proposal is reformulated to suit all clients.

Extract 2

```
01 SW1: voidaan esimerkiks tehdä vaikka joku kerta niin että
        we could for example at some point have

02      jokainen, (1.0) tekee vaikka oman cv:n [tai
        everybody (1.0) doing their own CV or so or

03 Pia:                                        [mul on
                                               [I have

04      valmiina jo kotona (0.2)
        my CV done at home (0.2)

05 SW1: ni,
        okay

06 Pia: se on ihan vähän aikaa sitte päivitetty
        I updated it quite recently

07 SW1: nii
        okay
08 Pia: se on ihan vähän aikaa sitte päivitetty.
        I updated it quite recently

09 SW1: hyvä (-)
        good (-)

10      (3.0)

11 SW1: mut onks tällaseen kiinnostusta vai onks se
        but are you interested in this thing or does it

12      tuntuuks se (.) kaukaiselta? (.) turhalta?
        does it feel (.) distant (.) unnecessary

13      (.) vaikeelta? [vai ihan hyvältä?
        (.) difficult or quite all right
```

14 Esa: [ihan hyvä ehdotus.
the suggestion is okay

15 (2.0)

16 SW2: mites Aki
how about Aki

17 Aki: siis ceeveen teko.
doing a CV you mean

18 SW2: mm

19 Aki: mul on mul on cv tehty.
I have I have done my CV

20 SW2: mm

21 Kia: mul ei
I haven't

22 (1.0)

23 SW1: sulhan on paljon työkokemusta.
you have a lot of work experience

24 SW2: mm,

((Kia tells about her work experience))

25 SW2: et mites sitte, (.) onks sitä koetteks te että
so what about this (.) is it do you think that it

26 siitä olis mitään hyötyä et käytäis niit läpi tai
would be useful at all to go through them or

27 jos haluis tuoda tänne että voitais yhdessä
if somebody would like to bring them here so we could

28 katto tai (0.2) vois esitellä muille et millasen
have a look together or (0.2) you could show

29 on tehny tai, (.) mitäs Pia (.) Aki on mieltä?
the CV you've done or (.) what do Pia (.) Aki think

30 (5.0)

31 SW1: oisko se ihan jees vai tuntuuks se (.) ei hyvältä
would it be ok or does it feel like (.)not a good

32 ajatukselta (.) esitellä omaa?
idea (.) to present your own

33 Pia: mä mietin sitä just (.) kais sen vois.
I was just thinking about it (.) I guess I could

34 SW1: mitkä fiilikset Akilla?
how do you feel Aki

35 (3.0)

36 Aki: oishan se,
it would be okay

37 (3.0)

38 SW2: mm. (.) must se ois ainaki mielenkiintoista
mm (.) at least I think it would be interesting

39 [että te voisitte kertoo sit vaik et miten te ootte
if you could tell then for example how you

40 Pia: [voin mä ottaa sen mukaan
yes I can bring it with me

41 SW2: tehny sen tai mistä te ootte saanu sen mallii ja
have done it or where you got the template and

42 (0.2) ootteko ite tehny vai saanu apua ja,
(0.2) did you do it yourself or did you get help and

43 Pia: mä sain äidiltä apua?
my mother helped me

44 SW2: nii
yes

45 SW1: nii ja sit vaikka esimerkiksi Kialla ei oo semmosta?
yes and even though Kia doesn't have a CV

46 Kia: mm-hm

47 SW1: ni sullakin on paljon työkokemusta niin sithän sä
you have a lot of work experience and then you would

48 saisit siitä hyvät (.) ehkä vinkkejä ja ideoita.
get good (.) perhaps some hints and ideas

49 Kia: mm

SW1 suggests drawing up a CV in a later meeting of the coaching group (lines 1–2). Pia answers by referring to the fact that she has a recently updated CV. Pia's turns (lines 3–4, 6, and 8) can be interpreted as an indirect rejection of the proposal: if she has a recently updated CV she is probably not interested in a future session of CV making. SW1 then asks the clients about their potential interest in the proposal (lines 11–13). Juha self-selects to give his support (line 14). SW2 asks Aki what he thinks about the proposal (line 16). In a similar way as Pia, Aki responds by referring to his existing CV (line 19), which indicates him declining the proposal.

At this point, Kia makes a remark about her lack of a CV (line 21). SW2 continues to reformulate the proposal, moving from suggesting that CVs be made, to using Pia and Aki's CVs as the basis for a group discussion (lines 25–29). The reformulation includes new elements that would also be acceptable and useful to Pia and Aki. The support workers explicitly ask Pia and Aki their opinions on the matter (lines 29, 31–32, 34). Although, neither of them express strong agreement, they do not oppose the proposal at this point (lines 33, 36). As the conversation moves on, SW1 underlines the benefits of the proposed activity from Kia's perspective (lines 45–48). Thus, the support workers use Kia's situation as a device for proceeding to acceptance of the proposal.

The clients in Extract 2 are explicitly encouraged to express their opinions on the proposed activity, and the disagreements are managed via the reformulation of the proposal to integrate different views into the outcome. Thus, the decision-making process has elements of deliberate consensus (Haug, 2015). However, most of the interactional work to achieve the decision is done by the support workers whereas the clients make comments from their own perspectives and do not actively take part in constructing a shared understanding among the whole group. Therefore, in this case, the consensus is not really the result of multilateral deliberation as such, but rather depends on the support workers' extensive use of inclusive practices.

Extract 3 illustrates another way of managing disagreements in a situation in which two clients are dominating the discussion. Previously the group had discussed the name of the group. Maj suggested "coaching group," whereas Anu and Leo promote the suggestion "work coaching group." The support workers ask the other clients for their opinions on the matter. The majority favor "work coaching group." In Extract 3, the support worker refers explicitly to the ideal of consensus to halt the acceptance of the decision in a situation where the divergent opinion of one client is in danger of being overlooked.

Extract 3

```
01 Leo: no ni. (.) mites me nyt päätämme tämän.
        well (.) how do we now make the decision

02 Anu: no enemmistö päätti sen (---)
        well the majority made the decision (---)

03      (.)

04 SW1: tai sitten me tehdään konsensus-päätös. heh heh heh
        or then we make a consensus decision heh heh heh heh

05      (.)

06 SW1: yksikin eriävä mielipide vaikuttaa. (.)
        even one dissenting opinion makes a difference (.)

07      meidän täytyy sit, (0.3) mi[ettiä
        we then have to (0.3) consider

08 Anu:                            [me ollaan sit ens viikolla
                                   then we're still next week

09      vielä tässä (---)
        here (---)

10      ((laughter))

11 SW1: ei se mitään meil on aik(h)aa.
        doesn't matter we have time

        ((Leo makes an assessment in order to support
         the name "work coaching group"))

12 Leo: et sen takia just ninku se että ku siinä on se
        so because of that the very thing that it includes
```

13 työvalmennus (.) niin se ↑itessään jo nimi
work coaching then the name in itself

14 kertoo (.) sen että mitä (.) mitä tää ninku
tells (.) what what (.) what this really

15 oikeen on.=mitä me täällä ninku puuhastellaan.
is that we're doing here

((Esa makes a new suggestion,"work group",
that causes joking and laughing))

16 SW2: okei?
okay

17 Leo: miksi me päätimme tämän.
what have we decided

18 Anu: laita se työvalmennus.
write down the work coaching

19 SW1: käyks se (.) käyks se kaikille.
is it (.) is it okay for everybody

20 Esa: eiks melkein kaikki sitä äänestäny.
didn't almost everyone vote for that option

21 SW1: no Maj ehdotti kyl toista ja mä: mullo kävi kaikki,
well Maj suggested something else and I'm okay with

22 (.) kaikki k(h)äy,
(.) everything

23 (2.0)

24 Anu: niin no se on nyt sittee se.
so well that's now what it is

```
25        (1.0)

26 Anu:   päätös tapahtu (--) demokratia (-) vai
          the decision was made (--) democracy (-) or

27        (3.0)

          ((Anu & Leo talk about the writing of the decision
            in the memo))

28 SW1:   pystyyks Maj elään sen ajatuksen kans jos me
          are you okay with it Maj, if we

29        otetaan toi (.) työvalmennusryhmä.
          choose that (.) work coaching group

30 Maj:   joo ihan hyvi:n,
          yes it's all right

31 SW1:   ei tule (.) @paha mieli@ ett(h)ä (.) <jyrättiin,>
          so you don't feel bad that we (.) overrode
```

In line 1, Leo refers to making a decision about something that needs to be done. However, Anu refers to the decision in the past tense, indicating the action being completed, and that the majority made the decision (line 2). At this point, SW1 makes an explicit reference to a consensus-based decision (line 4). A noticeable detail is that SW1's reference is followed by laughter, which can be interpreted as a way of relieving tension after disagreement (Wasson, 2016). SW1 continues, mentioning that the divergent opinion of just one client can count as reason to halt the process toward a majority-based decision (lines 6–7). Anu criticizes the prolonging of the decision-making process (lines 8–9), to which SW1 responds by underlining its unhurried pace (line 11).

After SW1 postpones the acceptance of the majority decision, Leo makes an assessment in support of the option "work coaching group" (lines 12–15). In line 17, Leo returns to the finalizing of the decision. Anu presents the name "work coaching group" as having been decided on (line 18). SW1 asks for acceptance from all the participants (line 19), and following Esa's account of majority support (line 20), once again notes one divergent opinion (line 21). As Anu strongly guides the interaction toward the finalization of the decision (lines 24, 26), SW1 explicitly asks Maj whether she would accept the decision which other clients favor (lines 28–29, 31).

Compared with Extract 2, in which the support workers reformulated the proposal to integrate the different views, the form of the proposal in Extract 3 could not be modified in a similar way because the choice was between specific options. However, the support worker takes responsibility for the management of one diverging opinion: she halts the interaction by referring explicitly to the ideal of consensus and allows the decision to be accepted only when no one opposes it.

The Retrospective Framing of Interaction

Besides framing the interaction prospectively, the support workers also framed it retrospectively as matching the ideal of consensus. Extract 4a features support worker SW1 summing up the decision-making process of considering an employee for Transitional Employment.

Extract 4a

```
01 SW1: ja sit me päädytään mun mielestä siihen ollaanko
        and then I guess we end up discussing whether we

02      samaa mieltä että ku (.) Aki itsevarmana miehenä (.)
        agree that when (.) Aki as a confident man (.)

03      paljo työkokemusta tehneenä
        with a lot of work experience

        ((omitted 6 lines: SW1 lists the strengths of Aki))

04 SW1: et kyl mä oikeen sanon et oot ahkera kaveri, .hh
        so I would say that you're a diligent guy .hh

05      niin voisko aatella et sä pistettäs kokeiltas tota
        so could we think that you we would try to
```

```
06        meiltä ensi tota Akia tyrkyttää sinne tota noin ni
          first push Aki from us to that place so

07        seuraavaan haastatteluun sitte (--) sitte ihmetellään
          then to the next interview then (--) then we wonder

08        että jos, (0.3) meilt on kolmesta näin hyvästä valittu
          if (0.3) we have chosen one of these three good ones

09        ni tota jos ei se pääse ni, (0.2)
          and if he isn't selected so (0.2)

10        mitäs meijän pitäis tehä. (0.2)
          what shall we do then (0.2)

11        että kyllä mä ninku (.) suosittelisin melkein
          so well I would (.) recommend pretty much

12        näitten keskustelujen pohjalta ihan tätä samaa.
          the same thing based on these discussions

13        (.)

14 SW1:   oltasko tyytyväisii jos tehtäs ny näin.
          are we satisfied if we do it like this now

15        (0.4)

16 SW1:   ei kellekään jääny semmosta tunnetta että ei ois
          so nobody got the feeling that he wasn't

17        otettu huomioon (0.5)
          given any attention (0.5)

18        huomioon on [((katsoo Juhaa ja nyökkää)) meinaan
          any attention((gazes Juha and nods)) I mean

19 Esa:               [((katsoo SW1:ta ja nyökkää takaisin))
                       ((gazes SW1 and nods))

20 SW1:   on otettu kaikki kyllä tosi hyvin.
          we have taken everything really well
```

SW1 initially frames her turn in terms of soliciting the group members' opinions by asking "do we agree" (lines 1–2). Then she describes Aki in a favorable light, mentioning his self-confidence and work experience (lines 2–3). SW1 continues to recommend Aki's choice. She continually uses the "we" form, indicating a joint decision. In lines 11–12, however, she uses the form "I would recommend pretty much", taking responsibility for the decision, although expressing it as a "recommendation".

In line 14, SW1 asks for the group's acceptance of the decision in the wording of the question "are we satisfied". When nobody responds, she produces a new turn (lines 16–17) in which she asks whether anybody felt he or she had not been noticed in the process. Next, SW1 makes the assessment (lines 18, 20) that everybody has really been heard, thereby indicating that her questioning of whether all views had been taken account was not really unnecessary. She also gazes at Esa and nods (line 18), which can be interpreted as an invitation for a confirming response from him. Esa responses with a slight nod (line 19).

The finalizing of the decision-making process in Extract 4a is led by the support worker. Although she explicitly asks for the group's opinion on the decision (line 14), and whether everybody is happy with the process (lines 16–17), her lexical choices imply a preference for consensual views, and makes the questioning of the upcoming decision difficult. Thus, the support worker articulates the decision, which can be considered to be *acclaimed consensus* (Haug, 2015).

Extract 4b is a continuation of the previous one. Here, the support worker explicitly asks the group to comment on the decision-making process.

Extract 4b

```
01 SW1: jees, (.) hyvä palaveri ihan älyttömän
        yes (.) a good meeting really

02      mielenkiintonen.
        interesting

03 Aki: jooh okeih
        yes okey

04 SW1: mitä, (.) käydään nopee kierros vielä et mitä
        what (.) let's take a last quick round so what

05      tää tämmönen tapa tuntuu käsitellä asioita.
        does this way of dealing with things feel like
        ((addressed to Lea))

06 Lea: ihan hyvältä.
        good.

07 SW1: joo, (.) ihan asiallista.
        yes (.) quite all right

08 Lea: joo.
        yes

        ((SW1 asks what Lea learned from the discussion))

09 SW1: no mites Aki miltä susta tuntuu tämmönen
        well Aki how do you feel about this

10      ku tällee yhdessä
        when we like do this together
```

```
11 Aki: öö:: kyllä on tämä hyvä haastattelu
        well this really is a good interview

        ((Aki tells his previous interview experiences))

12 SW1: mitä tämmönen tapa että me yhdessä
        how does this kind of convention of speaking

13      puhutaan täällä asioista
        together about things here

        miten koet tän ite. ((suunnattu Esalle))
        how do you feel about it ((to Esa))

14 Esa: oli musta ihan hyvä.
        I think it was good.

15 SW1: joo
        yes

        ((SW1 asks if Esa found any areas of development
          in himself))

16 SW1: mites Karo, ((työntekijä SW2))
        what do you think Karo ((support worker SW2))

17 SW2: mm-m? (.) tosi hyvä oli, (.) hyvä että
        mm (.) I think it was great (.) good that

18      päästiin tämmöseen ratkasuun.
        we ended up with this solution

19 SW1: tää on semmosta hommaa mitä varmaan joudutaan
        this is something that I guess
```

```
20    me kaikki tekee. (.) mä olin tässä nyt
      we all do (.) I was now
21    puheenjohtajana ja koko ajan äänessä ja vein tätä
      the chair and speaking all the time and in charge
22    mut Karo ja muutkin työntekijät
      but Karo and the other support workers
23    tekee tätä jatkossa et tällee käsitellään
      will do this in the future that we discuss
24    vaan yhdessä ja sovitaan asioita.
      and decide on matters together
```

SW1 invites everybody to comment on the decision-making process (lines 4–5). It is defined as a joint process, something the group members do "together" (lines 10, 12). Thus, the presupposition is that the process was implemented as a collective endeavor. One at a time, the clients describe the process as good (lines 6, 11, 14). SW2 makes an upgraded assessment by referring to the process as "great" (line 17). At the end of the segment, SW1 once again highlights the decision-making as something the participants do together (lines 23–24), while looking forward to similar, upcoming situations.

The support worker retrospectively frames the decision-making as consensus-based—even though she is in charge (see Extract 4a). In making an explicit reference to the social-communicative conventions of the Clubhouse community (line 12), she implies that the current process has fulfilled these very ideals. Consequently, focusing on the decision-making process means that the outcome and its basis are put to one side in the discussion.

Conclusions

The standards of the community-based Clubhouse model of mental health rehabilitation prescribe that decisions at the Clubhouse should be made by consensus. The findings from this study highlight the role of support workers' interactional practices in maintaining the ideological basis of the Clubhouse. Support workers draw on local contingencies to frame the situation prospectively as one that involves consensus-based decision-making (Extract 1). Additionally, when the decision has been established, support workers define the decision-making process leading up to it as a collective endeavor (Extracts 4a–4b) and initiate an evaluation round (Extract 4b) to frame the process retrospectively as matching the ideal of consensus. The study also reveals two ways of managing disagreements during the decision-making process to end up with consensus. When there are divergent opinions, support workers reconstruct the proposal to integrate the different views and ensure acceptance among the participants (Extract 2). However, when the decision should be made between specific options, meaning that the form of the proposal cannot easily be modified, decisions are made by the majority. In such cases, the support workers ensure that the disagreements are managed. Explicit references to the notion of consensus provide the support workers with a resource to halt the interaction in situations where discussion on divergent opinions is about to be silenced (Extract 3).

In our further discussion we start with the notion of deliberative consensus (Haug, 2015). This refers to decision-making processes in which participants are encouraged to express divergent views openly, the aim being to incorporate all views in a joint outcome. This resonates with Habermas's vision of the ideal speech situation, in which he defines consensus decision-making as a matter of authentic, inclusive, and respectful argumentation among participants who are motivated by the common good and who consider each other to be willing to reach a mutual understanding (Habermas, 1973). A prerequisite in the realization of deliberative consensus is a non-restrictive atmosphere throughout the decision-making process. This is a reflection of the notion that the process and outcome of deliberative consensus are closely connected, and experience of the process may sometimes be an even stronger determinant in the finalizing of the decision-making than the specific content of the outcome (Haug, 2015, p. 576). The ideal of consensus decision-making, through which the process and the outcome are interwoven, is in line with the guiding principles of the Clubhouse Community (Clubhouse International, 2019). However, the above analysis reveals some variation in emphasis between these two dimensions. In the case of prospective framing (Extract 1), the process and the outcome are presented in a causal relationship: if people participate in the forthcoming discussion, it will lead to a joint outcome that will suit everyone. However, given that achieving a joint outcome may not be possible in the real consensus-making situation, and that some participants must abandon their preferences (Extract 3), support workers turn to highlighting the experience of the process and try to ensure that it is positive for all, even if the outcome is not. Furthermore, as the examples of retrospective framing show (Extracts 4a–4b), when the outcome is led by a support worker acting alone, evaluation of the shared process is explicitly raised as a topic, whereas the outcome is not included in the discussion. Hence, the results from this study illustrate that, in the Clubhouse context, consensus-based decision-making refers above all to a shared decision-making process.

Another dimension worth discussing concerns the practices of support workers as exemplifying socialization. As argued above, the guiding principles in this type of community-based rehabilitation model cannot operate only at the level of professional practice, but all members of the community should be socialized into these conventions (Kaipio, 1999). Therefore, the actions of support workers referred to above serve not only to support clients locally during discussions, but also to grow clients into the social-communicative conventions of the Clubhouse. Moreover, the opportunity for clients to get involved in interactional situations that would not occur naturally, and to get support from support workers in managing these situations, could be considered an encouraging experience, which has reportedly improved clients' social relationships in private life (Carolan, Onaga, Pernice-Duca, & Jimenez, 2011).

Finally, we return to the consensus-making process and the outcome. As we have argued, consensus decision-making in the Clubhouse context appears to be specifically about the shared process, in which support workers use various means to promote the participation of clients, whereas the actual outcome might be the achievement of a few that others just accept. Inequalities in the resources of participants, such as argumentation skills and social status, have a major impact, especially on the determination of consensus—the ability to further one's own preferences is crucial in this type of decision-making (Urfalino, 2014, p. 339). Thus, consensus-based decision-making is not a synonym for democratic decision-making. Therefore, the question is whether it is applicable in all cases, or whether some issues should be decided by means of majority voting (cf. Rae, 1969), meaning that each participant has equal weight in the outcome.

References

Bohman, J. (1996). *Public deliberation: Pluralism, complexity, and democracy.* Cambridge, MA: MIT Press.

Carolan, M., Onaga, E., Pernice-Duca, F., & Jimenez, T. (2011). A place to be: The role of clubhouses in facilitating social support. *Psychiatric Rehabilitation Journal, 35*(2), 125–132.

Clubhouse International. (2019). *Quality standards.* http://clubhouse-intl.org.

De Leon, G. (2000). *The therapeutic community: Theory, model, and method.* New York, NY: Springer.

Haapamäki, J., Kaipio, K., Keskinen, S., Uusitalo, I., & Kuoksa, M. (2000). *Päivähoito oppimis- ja kasvatusyhteisönä* [Day-care as a learning and educational community]. Helsinki: Tammi.

Habermas, J. (1973). Wahrheitstheorien. In H. Fahrenbach (Ed.), *Wirklichkeit und Reflexion. Walter Schulz zum 60. Geburtstag* (pp. 211–265). Pfullingen: Neske.

Habermas, J. (1981). *Theorie des Kommukativen Handelns. Band 1. Handlungsrationalität und gesellschaftliche Rationalisierung.* Frankfurt am Main: Suhrkamp Verlag.

Habermas, J. (1988). *Theorie des Kommukativen Handelns. Band 2. Zur Kritik der funktionalistischen Vernunft.* Frankfurt am Main: Suhrkamp Verlag.

Hänninen, E. (2012). *Choices for recovery: Community-based rehabilitation and the Clubhouse model as means to mental health reforms.* Helsinki: Finnish Institute for Health and Welfare.

Haug, C. (2015). What is consensus and how is it achieved in meetings? Four types of consensus decision-making. In J. A. Allen, N. Lehmann-Willenbrock, & S. G. Rogelberg (Eds.), *The Cambridge handbook of meeting science* (pp. 556–584). Cambridge: Cambridge University Press.

Jones, I. R. (2001). Habermas or Foucault or Habermas and Foucault? The implications of a shifting debate for medical sociology In G. Scambler (Ed.), *Habermas critical theory and health* (pp. 163–181). London: Routledge.

Kaipio, K. (1999). *Kasvattava yhteisö* [Educational community]. Jyväskylä: Gummerus.

Lawson, M. A. (2016). The healing nature of communion: Scottish psychoanalysis, RD Laing, and therapeutic communities. *Journal of Theoretical and Philosophical Psychology, 36*(1), 20–28.

Oshima, S. (2014). Achieving consensus through professionalized head nods: The role of nodding in service encounters in Japan. *International Journal of Business Communication, 51*(1), 31–57.

Rae, D. (1969). Decision rules and individual values in constitutional choice. *American Political Science Review, 63*(1), 40–56.

Scambler, G. (2001). Introduction: Unfolding themes of an incomplete project. In G. Scambler (Ed.), *Habermas, critical theory, and health* (pp. 1–24). London: Routledge.

Scheff, T. J. (1967). Toward a sociological model of consensus. *American Sociological Review, 32*(1), 32–46.

Schegloff, E. A. (2007). *Sequence organization in interaction: A primer in conversation analysis*. Cambridge: Cambridge University Press.

Sidnell, J., & Stivers, T. (2013). *The handbook of conversation analysis*. Boston, MA: Wiley-Blackwell.

Stolte, J. F., Fine, G. A., & Cook, K. S. (2001). Sociological miniaturism: Seeing the big through the small in social psychology. *Annual Review of Sociology, 27*, 387–413.

Tanaka, K., Craig, T., & Davidson, L. (2016). Clubhouse community support for life: Staff–member relationships and recovery. *Journal of Psychosocial Rehabilitation and Mental Health, 2*(2), 131–141.

Tanaka, K., & Davidson, L. (2015). Meanings associated with the core component of clubhouse life: The work-ordered day. *Psychiatric Quarterly, 86*(2), 269–283.

Urfalino, P. (2014). The rule of non-opposition: Opening up decision-making by consensus. *Journal of Political Philosophy, 22*(3), 320–341.
Walker, P., & Lovat, T. (2016). Dialogic consensus in clinical decision-making. *Journal of Bioethical Inquiry, 13*, 571–580.
Wasson, C. (2016). Integrating conversation analysis and issue framing to illuminate collaborative decision-making activities. *Discourse & Communication, 10*(4), 378–411.

Index

C. Lindholm et al. (eds.), *Joint Decision Making in Mental Health*, The Language of Mental Health, https://doi.org/10.1007/978-3-030-43531-8

The manufacturer's authorised representative in the EU is Springer Nature Customer Service Centre GmbH, Europaplatz 3, 69115 Heidelberg, Germany. If you have any concerns regarding our products, please contact ProductSafety@springernature.com

Printed and bound by CPI Group (UK) Ltd, Croydon, CR0 4YY
30/09/2026
02225461-0013